RIGHT · LEFT
BRAIN · BRAIN

REFLEXOLOGY

RIGHT LEFT BRAIN BRAIN

REFLEXOLOGY

A Self-help Approach to
Balancing Life's Energies with Color,
Sound, and Pressure-Point Techniques

Madeleine Turgeon, N.D.

Translated by Marie-Andrée Guoin

Healing Arts Press
Rochester, Vermont

Healing Arts Press
One Park Street
Rochester, Vermont 05767

First published in French under the title *La réflexologie du cerveau pour auditifs et visuels* by Editions de Mortagne, Quebec, 1988

First U.S. edition 1994 by Healing Arts Press

Note to the reader: This book is intended as an informational guide. The remedies, approaches, and techniques described herein are meant to supplement, and not to be a substitute for, professional medical care or treatment. They should not be used to treat a serious ailment without prior consultation with a qualified healthcare professional.

Library of Congress Cataloging-in-Publication Data

Turgeon, Madeleine.
    [Réflexologie du cerveau pour auditifs et visuels. English]
    Right-brain left-brain reflexology : a self-help approach to balancing life's energies with color, sound, and pressure-point techniques / Madeleine Turgeon.
1st U.S. ed.
        p.   cm
    Includes index.
    ISBN 0-89281-432-2
    1. Reflexotherapy. 2. Cerebral dominance. I. Title.
RM723.R43T8713   1993
615.8'22—dc20   93-6778
                                                                              CIP

Printed and bound in the United States

10 9 8 7 6 5 4 3 2 1

Text design by Charlotte Tyler

Healing Arts Press is a division of Inner Traditions International

Distributed to the book trade in the United States by American International Distribution Corporation (AIDC)

Distributed to the book trade in Canada by Publishers Group West, (PGW), Montreal West, Quebec

Contents

Introduction

A Dialogue Between the Hemispheres of the Brain

One evening a man named Ananda was looking for something on the ground, near a streetlight, when a friend passed by.

"Did you lose something, Ananda?" asked the friend.

"Yes, I lost my key," replied Ananda.

And so the friend bent over and together they looked for the key. After a time, the friend spoke up. "Where exactly did you lose it?" he asked.

"At home," Ananda answered.

"But Ananda, why are you looking for it here?" his friend exclaimed.

"Because there's more light here!" Ananda replied.

This story might seem amusing or foolish to you. How could one possibly find a key lost in a dark house by looking outside under a street lamp? It does not make sense! The rational, linear mind feels certain that this search is useless. And yet, how often do we oversimplify, ignoring important but confusing factors in an effort to "shed more light" on a subject and, in doing so, lose sight of the dark, ambiguous mystery where the misplaced key really lies?

We all have these two sides to ourselves: a logical, rational side,

1

associated with the left hemisphere of the brain, which enjoys clarity and can formulate explicit thoughts; and a more mysterious side, the right hemisphere, which is at home in complexity and ambiguity, darkness and subtlety, and can intuitively grasp truths that the left brain does not recognize.

Each of us is born with a predilection for perceiving and responding to the world from one hemisphere of the brain. Yet the extent to which we can mobilize our *nondominant* hemisphere determines our state of overall physical and mental well-being. In this book I aim to help you identify your dominant brain hemisphere and use that knowledge to practice specific techniques for correcting energy imbalances in the body, thereby inviting a free flow of communication between the two hemispheres.

My training in the healing arts began with the study of pressure-point reflexology. Based on theories introduced by two American doctors early in the twentieth century,[1] reflexology is a method of massaging certain points on the hands and feet in order to affect the health of the whole body by restoring the balance of vital energy and improving circulation. The points chosen in a reflexology massage are those that have a reflex connection to other areas of the body. Characteristic of reflexology are its charts of correspondences between points on the hands and feet and the vital organs of the body these reflex points govern.

The modern science of holography provides a sophisticated explanation for the effectiveness of traditional reflexology. Holography posits the hologram as a new principle of the organization of matter. In a hologram, all the information about an entire object is stored in each one of its points. If the hologram is broken, each of the pieces holds the information required to reconstruct the whole picture. Some well-known scientists contend that the brain—indeed the whole universe—has holographic properties. This modern notion of a holographic universe is compatible with mystical experience. Witness Blake's ". . . to see the world in a grain of sand . . ." Another description of the holographic perspective can be found in a Hindu sutra: "It is said that there is, in the Indra Heaven, a

---

1. In 1913 Dr. William Fitzgerald and Dr. Edwin F. Bowers outlined the basis of reflexology. Subsequently two women, Eunice D. Ingham and Mildred Carter, worked to further promote reflexology, with Kevin and Barbara Kunz also contributing significantly to its rapid spread.

trellis of pearls set in such a way that when you look at one, you see the reflections of all the others." In this holographic perspective, each object in the world is not only itself but encompasses all others.

The holographic theory supports the basic concept of reflexology: that the hand and foot (and other parts of the body) form a microcosm of the whole body and can thus influence any of its organs. Indeed, one can also affect the systems of the body by working from the nose (sympathicotherapy), the eye (iridology), the ear (auriculotherapy), the tongue, and, of course, the brain itself.

How This Book Came To Be Written

In 1980 I published my first book on reflexology entitled *Découvrons la Réflexologie*[2] *(Discovering Reflexology),* and in 1985 I published a second book, *Energie et Réflexologie*[3] *(Energy and Reflexology).* Both books address the subject of hand and foot reflexology as well as the basic concepts of energy polarity. I was encouraged to write this present book in attempting to answer an apparently simple question asked in one of my workshops. The question was "How can you practice reflexology in a way that accounts for the polarity between the two sides of the brain?"

I was unable to come up with an answer at the time and realized that as far as the relationship between reflexology and the hemispheres of the brain was concerned, my own mind was in darkness rather than in light. So began the journey that led to the writing of this book.

I began my explorations with a basic understanding of the anatomy and physiology of the brain acquired in college and then furthered my study independently. The intellectual knowledge (left hemisphere) I acquired was, however, virtually useless in daily life. The left brain may find comfort in knowing certain terms such as *rhombencephalon* (hindbrain) or *prosencephalon* (forebrain), but the left brain was not helping me to understand or integrate this information. How could I get out of the left brain and into the right? How could I truly get in touch with this information?

---

2. Madeleine Turgeon, *Découvrons la Réflexologie* (Ottawa, Canada: Les Editions de Mortagne, 1980).
3. Madeleine Turgeon, *Energie et Réflexologie* (Ottawa, Canada: Les Editions de Mortagne, 1985).

"Seek, and ye shall find; knock, and the door shall be opened!" One day, while working through the exercises in a book entitled *Drawing on the Right Side of the Brain*,[4] I experienced a dramatic change in consciousness. I felt my energy suddenly shift from the left side of my brain to the right, and in that moment I discovered an unsuspected talent—I could draw! This new reality seemed so simple, so obvious, that it was as if I had always known it, although moments before I couldn't draw a thing. My right brain had been activated—I had left the zone of the left brain, illuminated by the streetlight, to enter the dark house where the key lay, a world full of promise and fabulous treasure.

This discovery made me very aware of the reality and importance of the two hemispheres of the brain. The sudden experience of the holistic, relational capacities of the right brain was a revelation to my linear, rational left brain. I realized how important it is for all of us to know which hemisphere is dominant and to gain access to our nondominant, hidden side.

This experience spurred me on in my research. I gathered information from many different sources and was immensely helped by a collection of notes on the hemispheres of the brain published by Ivon Robert,[5] a professor at the CEGEP du Vieux Montréal. I also came across the work of Dr. Raymond Lafontaine,[6] a pediatric neurologist from Montreal. In the 1960s Dr. Lafontaine developed a theory about auditory and visual information processing. In his clinical practice he observed that people process information in two very different ways: he classified these two types of people as *auditories*—those who rely on sound for information processing, and *visuals*—those who understand information relative to what they see. Through my own research I came to realize that these typologies could also be classified as *right-brain dominant* and *left-brain*

---

4. Betty Edwards, *Drawing on the Right Side of the Brain* (Los Angeles: J. P. Tarcher, Inc., 1979).

5. "La Pédagogie Des Visuel-les et Des Auditif-ves," 1982 and "La Pédagogie Des Visuelles et Des Auditif-ves: Applications Pratiques," 1984 (Montreal: CEGEP du Vieux Montréal, Department of Psychology). See also Ivon Robert, *Auditif-ves, visuel-les, audiovisuel-les* (Montreal: Editions Ivon Robert, 1985).

6. Dr. Raymond Lafontaine and Béatrice Lessoil, *Etes-vous auditif ou visuel?* (Verriers, Belgium: S.A. Les Nouvelles Editions Marabout, 1984) and *L'Univers des auditifs et des visuels* (Quebec: Les Editions du Nouveau Monde, Inc., 1981). See also Ghislane Meunier-Tardif, *Les auditifs et les visuels: le principe de Lafontaine* (Canada: Linre Expression, 1985).

dominant, respectively, as their profiles were in such accord. This understanding was key to learning how to apply healing techniques according to the hemispheric dominance of the receiver.

Beyond Touch

In 1973, through my study of naturopathy, I came into contact with color healing (chromotherapy) and in particular with the work of Linda Clark, who promotes the practice of color breathing. At the time I did not really understand how one could breathe colors, so I dismissed the idea until I became acquainted with the world of auditories and visuals and their fundamentally different approaches to life. I realized then that I needed to go beyond the concept of simply touching a reflex point with my fingers in order to stimulate healing. Through my own experience and practice I had come to know that there are two types of touch: that which originates on the outside, when my hand or body touches an external object; and that which originates on the inside, in the mind, as when I *imagine* a touch or other sensory experience. These two ways of working are integrally connected: in the practice of holographic medicine, any action we perform on one part of the being reacts throughout the whole being. By touching the body at the skin level, on the reflex points, we touch the mind, and by contacting the mind with colors or sounds, we touch the body. Using this "internal touch," we can deeply influence our own systems without the need for someone to actually lay hands on us. My introduction to the auditory and visual typologies and their different means of processing information brought forth the realization that the internal practice of color breathing could be used to activate *one's own* reflex points, and that the particulars of the practice were determined by the dominant brain hemisphere. Through this practice one can release energies trapped in the dominant brain, thereby creating a clear pathway for communication between the hemispheres. This increased communication provides access to the nondominant hemisphere and so opens a vast wellspring of energy and potential.

Chinese Medicine, Sound, and Color

As I had already been working extensively on integrating the ancient wisdom of Traditional Chinese Medicine with the newer techniques of reflexology, I used my knowledge of the Chinese Law of Five Elements as my guide in determining what colors auditories and visuals should breathe. This will be further discussed in chapter five. As I began introducing this technique to my clients I was amazed to find that those who practiced it not only experienced a significant reduction in discomfort, but often saw their pain disappear instantaneously. Color reflexology had just been born! Over the following weeks, however, I came to realize that visuals were having greater results than auditories. At that point it did not take much to conjecture that reflexology using sound would be better suited to auditories. This notion was easy to implement, since Chinese tradition associates specific musical notes with each of the five elements. And so it was that sound reflexology became the harmonious complement to color reflexology.

I invite you now to explore these discoveries with me. I recommend that you breathe slowly and deeply as you read to assist in making this a full-body experience.

The first chapter of *Right-Brain Left-Brain Reflexology* covers basic information on the structure and function of the brain. Chapter two explains in detail the functions of the two cerebral hemispheres and the characteristics of people with left- or right-hemispheric dominance. Chapter three describes the classifications of auditory and visual and presents a questionnaire and other tools that will help you determine your type. Chapter four details the all-important methods for switching hemispheres and balancing the two sides of the brain.

The last four chapters present specific reflexology techniques. In chapter five I describe the practice of color and sound reflexology, tracing the roots of this practice to the Hindu chakra system and the Chinese Law of Five Elements and explaining how it can be best employed to heal conditions of dis-ease in modern Western man. Chapter six provides guidance for the practice of auriculotherapy (ear reflexology), an ancient healing practice made more accessible by taking hemispheric dominance into consideration. The systems charts in chapter seven outline the steps to follow in applying color and sound reflexology and auriculotherapy to support the healing of various physical conditions. Chapter eight gives instructions on a practice for harmonizing the energy channels of the body in order to eliminate phobias and balance the emotions.

My purpose in writing this book is to help you maintain a healthy, happy dialogue between the two sides of your brain so that you may live more harmoniously with yourself and others.

1

The Three Biological Computers

It is curious that one is required to have a license to operate an automobile but not to operate the brain, a much more complicated device that nevertheless works according to relatively simple principles. An understanding of the triune brain and how it functions allows us to use the brain much more effectively.

The well-known neuroscientist P. D. McLean explains that the brain is a triune structure (figure 1) composed of three distinct biological computers, each having its own unique intelligence, sense of time and space, memory, and motor functions.[7] These three parts are called the *reptilian complex,* the *limbic system,* and the *neocortex.*

The Reptilian Complex

The reptilian complex (figure 2) includes the cerebellum; the brainstem, composed of the medulla oblongata, the pons, and the mesencephalon; and the diencephalon, composed of the pineal and pituitary glands, thalamus, hypothalamus, and optic nerves. This, the primitive part of the brain, is the portion we share with the reptiles. It is the seat of these activities:

---

7. See P. D. McLean, "The Triune Brain: Emotion and Scientific Bias" in F. O. Schmit (ed.), *The Neurosciences, Second Study Program* (New York: Rockefeller University Press, 1970).

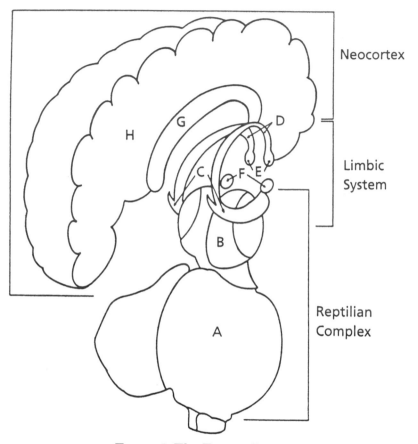

FIGURE 1: The Triune Brain

A. Cerebellum
B. Brain stem
C. Hippocampal gyrus
   and fimbria
D. Septum
E. Mammillary bodies
F. Amygdaloid bodies
G. Corpus callosum
H. Left hemisphere

- Regulation of all vital functions, including heartbeat, blood pressure and circulation, breathing, digestion, fluctuations in body temperature, the waking/sleeping/dreaming cycle, and endocrine system responses.
- Automatic and instinctive reactions such as hunger, thirst, survival, sexual activity, fertility, and lactation.
- Selective concentration: the filtering of sensory messages going to the higher levels of the brain.

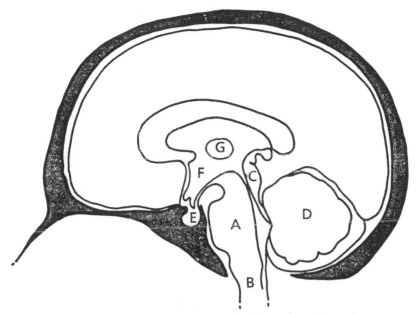

FIGURE 2: Structure of the Reptilian Complex

A. Pons
B. Medulla oblongata
C. Mesencephalon (mid brain)
D. Cerebellum

E. Pituitary gland (hypophysis)
F. Hypothalamus
G. Thalamus
A + B + C: Brain stem or reticular system

- Coordination of muscular activity as a whole, including balance, sense of position, muscle tone, and fine motor control.
- Motivation and drive, including reactions to stress and fear, due to the pleasure/pain centers located in the hypothalamus.
- Sensory switching station—the thalamus receives all incoming sensory information and routes it to the specific sensory areas (visual, auditory, olfactory, etc.) of the higher brain.
- Presumably the seat of certain social behaviors such as imitation, territoriality, establishment of social hierarchies, and ritual making, as well as mating habits, feeding habits, and repetitive behaviors.

The reptilian brain is constantly informed about the physical state of the organism, and when necessary it transmits this information to the other parts of the brain. It is the representative of the body in the brain, the voice that presents the biological arguments in any course of action

9

It is, however, very limited in its ability to learn and respond to varying conditions, being confined to genetically programmed behavior patterns.

The Limbic System

Evolutionarily, the limbic system (figure 3) is a more recent part of the brain and is found in all mammals, reaching its fullest development in primates. The limbic system in a human brain weighs about three-quarters of a pound; it sits like a cap on top of the more primitive reptilian brain. It is directly connected to the cerebral cortex and to the hypothalamus, and indirectly to all sensory input. It includes the septum and septal region, the amygdala, the mammillary bodies, and the hippocampal gyrus and fimbria. It has two important functions:

- It is a selector, choosing from the environment whatever is appropriate to satisfy the needs of the organism. For instance, say you are outside in the sun, hot and thirsty, and have peanuts, dates, and water beside you. Without going through a conscious thought process you will choose to ingest the water first. This is the limbic system functioning. It has a lot to do with the likes and dislikes that are based on past experience. This brings us to the second major function of the limbic system.

- It is the physical core of our memory. The limbic system records information based on the strength of the emotion or sensation felt at the time of an experience. For example, you will have trouble remembering what you did a week ago if your activities were commonplace; however, you will very clearly recall a special evening spent with a friend a few months ago. The limbic system remembers pleasant and unpleasant experiences, successes and failures, as a guide for present-moment action.

The criteria for selecting and memorizing are different for the two sides of the brain. Being more action oriented, the left side of the brain is primarily involved with the muscular system and is strongly motivated by the emotions. The right side, being more receptive, is in greater contact with the senses and therefore more influenced by sensations.

The limbic system is involved in every step of information processing, including the selection of information, evaluating information in the

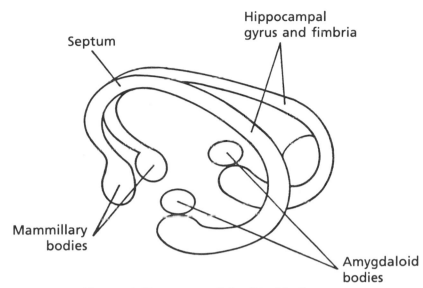

Septum

Hippocampal gyrus and fimbria

Mammillary bodies

Amygdaloid bodies

FIGURE 3: Structure of the Limbic System

light of past experience, motivating action, and remembering the results as successes or failures for future reference. While giving us the ability to learn from experience, in order to analyze and understand its environment the limbic system is largely dependent on the interpretation of events made by the neocortex.

The Neocortex

In evolutionary terms the neocortex is the most recent part of the brain. It appears in rudimentary form in the lower mammals and reaches full development in humans. The word *cortex* comes from the Latin *corium,* meaning "skin." The neocortex spreads out and wraps around the two more primitive brains; it occupies 85 percent of the volume of the brain and is made up of more than ten billion neurons (nerve cells), each having more than one hundred thousand connections with other neurons. It weighs about two and one-half pounds.

The neocortex has three important functions:

- Memory storage—experiences selected by the limbic system are stored biochemically in the neurons of the neocortex.

- Thinking and reasoning—thinking is made possible by extensive connections between neurons that enable associations to be made among facts stored in the memory.

- Sensory perception and motor control—the neocortex acts as the supervisor of sensory and motor function in the reptilian and limbic systems; it is also responsible for conscious control of movement and detailed conscious perception.

The neocortex is separated into a left and a right hemisphere. In lower mammals both hemispheres function in the same way, enabling the animal to have a social life and to communicate by signals and sounds. In humans, however, the hemispheres have taken on different but complementary functions, with each hemisphere having its own particular form of communication, memory, and information processing. The left hemisphere is analytical, specializing in the complex functions of reading, writing, speaking, counting, assessing details, and establishing cause-and-effect relations. It is the hemisphere that governs logical and abstract thinking. It controls the right side of the body. The right hemisphere is systemic. It allows us to comprehend a situation globally, to perceive it as a whole, and to assign a sensory charge to it. The right hemisphere governs empirical thinking. It controls the left side of the body. **The two hemispheres are of equal importance and complement one another.** They are joined by the corpus callosum, which allows them to communicate and to coordinate their functions.

Each part of the brain brings its own special capacities to the service of the same basic imperatives: to satisfy our needs, deal with the dangers of our environment, adapt to changing conditions, act in order to constantly improve our situations, and to benefit from all experiences.

In summary, we have three biological computers: the reptilian complex, which integrates physiological data; the limbic system, which integrates emotional data; and the neocortex, which integrates intellectual data (figure 4). Information enters the limbic system (1), which directs it to the right and left hemispheres of the neocortex (2). The information goes back and forth between the hemispheres via the corpus callosum (3), and gives rise to action if the emotional charge is sufficient (4). Reactions are provoked in the body (5). The experience is memorized by the limbic system (6).

Constant and unobscured communication between the two hemispheres of the brain is necessary if we are to make decisions appropriate

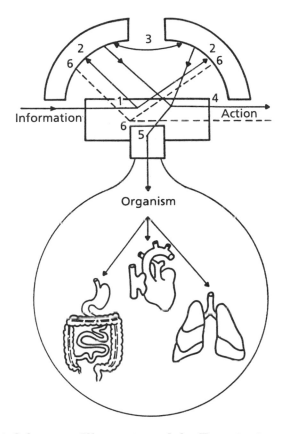

FIGURE 4: Schematic Illustration of the Functioning of the Brain

to the shifting circumstances of our lives. Some situations require immediate action; others require pondering and discussion before movement. The key is this: the better *each* hemisphere plays its role, the more effectively we can think, speak, and act in all situations.

2

The Left and Right
Hemispheres of the Brain

Before we take a more detailed look at the respective functions of the left
and right hemispheres, here are some interesting figures on the human
brain.

- The first vertebrate to have a brain appeared about four hundred and fifty million years ago. The human brain itself covers roughly one-tenth of biological time; i.e., it is forty-five
  million years old. Weighing approximately three pounds, it
  accounts for only two percent of the total body weight but
  consumes twenty percent of the oxygen supply (fifty percent
  in children). One-fifth of the body's blood flows through the
  brain, about one and one-half pints per minute.

- Neurons depend almost entirely on the energy provided by
  blood sugar. Sugar reserves stored in the brain are rather
  modest; if the blood flow is interrupted, the brain loses consciousness within a few seconds and starts to deteriorate within
  a few minutes.

- The surface of the two hemispheres is called the cortex. It is
  about one-eighth of an inch thick and contains at least ten
  billion (10^{10}) neurons—some estimate as much as ten times
  this amount. Each cell connects with at least six hundred
  other cells. The brain has an information storage capacity of

14

at least 10^{10} kilobytes, the equivalent of ten thousand encyclopedias. It radiates the same amount of energy as a twenty-five-watt light bulb.

General Characteristics of the Hemispheres

As we have already noted, the neocortex is divided into two interconnected hemispheres with complementary functions. The left hemisphere is analytical, breaking things down into separate parts in order to understand the whole, while the right hemisphere is systemic, grasping the whole system at once and making sense of the parts within this overall context.

This is a fundamental difference. The analytic approach presupposes a static view of life and provides the basis for the accumulation of knowledge, while the systemic approach offers a more dynamic view of life and supports inventive thinking. The two forms of thinking and conceiving work together, giving rise to all the achievements of the human mind.

To live a well-balanced life we need to make full use of both sides of the brain. However, each of us has a predisposition to one side or the other and may lack an understanding of the potentials inherent in the nondominant side. It is therefore very useful to gain a clear sense of the different yet complementary attributes of the two hemispheres, so that you can tell which is your dominant side and recognize the characteristics of the nondominant hemisphere that you may want to develop in your life. What follows is a detailed explanation of the overall characteristics of the two hemispheres. Later in the chapter we will look at how these characteristics are manifested in specific areas of behavior, and finally we will examine the attributes of people in whom one hemisphere strongly dominates the other.

The left brain breaks a whole into its basic components to grasp the nature of their relation and interaction. In order to do so, it reviews each element and retains those it feels are important. Thus, it can act on each of them and alter them as needed. This tendency of the left brain to focus mainly on details that have emotional impact often results in a loss of objectivity and to some extent isolates it from reality. This concern for detail leads the left brain to develop very precise plans that are generally difficult to apply because they suggest a rigid course of action that cannot adapt to life's ever-changing conditions.

The left brain is the action brain—it does not seek to know the reasons driving it toward a goal, only how to get there. To this end it proceeds by trial and error, checking out the validity of its theories in actual practice and experimenting until it has obtained the desired results. It is the theoretical practitioner.

The right brain has an overview of things. It relates events to each other and studies the effects of their interaction. It can act on a group of variables at the same time in order to achieve its objective. If the objective is long term, it will not easily give up. It has great perseverance.

Since the right brain views an issue as a whole, it develops the broad outlines of a plan after having first set very specific objectives. This plan is flexible and can be adapted to all types of situations. However, it checks the action model against reality before applying the plan. It therefore relies on experience before heading into the unknown. It is the practical theorist.

In short, the left brain manages short-term projects, isolates components, develops detailed plans (the "how"), and moves from the abstract to the concrete. The right brain, on the other hand, has an overall view of things, sets specific objectives (the "why"), and moves from the concrete to the abstract.

Specific Functions
of the Cerebral Hemispheres

We now turn to an examination of how these general characteristics manifest themselves in the way each hemisphere handles aspects of mental functioning. Each hemisphere has its own particular language, memory capacity, emotional tone, area of competence, cognitive process, and perceptual method. It bears repeating that the left and right hemispheres of the brain complement each other harmoniously. To effectively and effortlessly use both sides of your brain you must know their specific functions. This will be of considerable help in achieving your objectives.

The left brain is the center for abstract thought. It isolates the elements of a whole and analyzes them in sequential, linear fashion. It is a smooth talker. It has a verbal memory (for words and numbers) as well as an encyclopedic memory (for acquired knowledge). This acquired knowledge provides its basis for reasoning. On an abstract level, the left brain is logical and has accurate reasoning and sound judgment. It is gifted in

SUMMARY CHART[8]

GENERAL CHARACTERISTICS OF THE HEMISPHERES

LEFT BRAIN	RIGHT BRAIN
Analytical approach	Systemic approach

OVERALL STRATEGY

• Isolates/separates elements	• Links elements to each other, unites them
• Tries to determine the nature of the interaction between elements	• Tries to determine the effects over time of the interaction between elements
• Acts on one variable at a time	• Acts on many variables at once

OBJECTIVES

• To produce a detailed theory, often difficult to translate into action	• To produce a general model that may not be stringent but is nevertheless effective in action
• Action is preprogrammed in detail	• Action is based on objectives
• Knowledge of the means, the "how"	• Knowledge of the objectives, the "why"
• To support accumulation of knowledge	• To support creative thought

VALIDATION METHOD

• The experimental method: trial and error	• Modeling: direct comparison of the model with reality

languages and the exact sciences. Since it grasps things by analyzing them, it needs time to develop an overall view of a complex spatial structure. For this reason the left brain is said to be temporal.

At ease in the intellectual world, it is much less comfortable dealing with the myriad aspects of life that constitute reality. When assessing a

---

8. Chart inspired by Ivon Robert, *La pédagogie des visuel(les) et des auditifs(ves)* (*The Pedagogy of Visuals and Auditories*) (Montreal: Editions Ivon Robert, 1982) and by Joël De Rosnay, *Le macroscope* (*The Macroscope*) (Paris: Seuil, 1975.)

given situation the left-brain person will logically determine what will be the expected progression of events, analyzing all the known details in order to successfully accomplish his goal. Life can become very frustrating; indeed, he can even become paralyzed in his ability to take action, when unpredicted variables enter the situation and change its preconceived profile. The individual whose left brain is dominant tends to become discouraged when he fails. He needs to be reassured, to feel loved, hence his extroversion. This extroversion manifests itself through cheerfulness, optimism, and great sociability.

The right brain is the center for concrete thought. It supports its thinking with actual experience and uses a collection of images taken from that experience. It proceeds by analogy, by the association of ideas. Its perception is holistic. Generally speaking, words do not come easily to it. The right brain communicates through the arts (music, painting, sculpture, dance, etc.), at which it is particularly gifted. To express itself, the right brain uses speech full of images, often delivered in a monotone.

The memory system of the right brain deals with concrete experiences and individual phenomena. Its universe consists of images, symbols, and feelings relating to real-life experiences. The practice of resourcing from past experiences makes the right brain tend toward introversion and reflection. For this reason, the right-brain-dominant individual doesn't feel the need to be an extrovert. The approach of the right brain is systemic, giving it an overall perception of complex spatial structures and enabling it to identify a whole almost instantly from one of its basic elements. Thus the right brain is said to be timeless.

Characteristics of Hemispheric Dominance

The left and right hemispheres of the brain do not exist alone, without their other-hemisphere complement. Yet every day we encounter individuals who act predominantly from one hemisphere. Some people are adept at balancing this one-sidedness by activating the nondominant hemisphere, whereas others may be ruled almost entirely by their dominant side. To help bring this investigation closer to home, we will now discuss the various characteristics of people having one hemisphere that strongly dominates the other. Of necessity, we will draw something of a caricature in this discussion of "pure types." Characteristics from both typologies appear to a greater or lesser degree in all people, depending on their ability to invoke the nondominant hemisphere.

18

SUMMARY CHART

SPECIFIC FUNCTIONS OF THE CEREBRAL HEMISPHERES

LEFT BRAIN	RIGHT BRAIN
LANGUAGE	
• Abstract thought (knowledge) characterized by logical process employing concepts, words, and numbers • Facility for speaking	• Concrete thought characterized by symbolic and metaphorical images gathered from experience • Facility for music-making
MEMORY	
• Verbal memory characterized by concepts; encyclopedic knowledge	• Memory of phenomena/ specific experiences; feelings
EMOTIONAL TONE	
• Extrovert, characterized by optimism, sociability, cheerfulness	• Introvert, characterized by wisdom, reserve, seriousness
AREAS OF COMPETENCE	
• Reasoning—working from acquired knowledge • Language • Exact sciences (life sciences, mathematics, etc.)	• Reflection supported by actual experience • Art • Humanities (behavioral and social sciences, psychology, etc.)
COGNITIVE PROCESS	
• Secondary (temporal)—putting together pieces of a puzzle to come up with a general picture	• Primary (timeless)—immediate identification of a whole from one of its basic elements
PERCEPTUAL METHOD	
• Gradual perception of the elements of complex spatial structure	• Direct grasp of whole pattern of complex spatial structures

19

Left-brain- and right-brain-dominant people differ widely in their modes of cognitive functioning and even in the workings of their nervous systems. Relying on acquired knowledge, the left-brain-dominant person must test every aspect of a theory to ascertain its validity. He has an underinclusive mind that carefully reviews each element of a whole. His selective attention is narrow, specific, and intensive, and he can fail to see the obvious because of his concentration on details. You could say that the left-brain-dominant person can't see the forest for the trees.

On a neurophysiological level, he has what could be called a tense or agitated nervous system. That is, he has little capacity for self-restraint, tending to overreact to incoming stimuli. He must thus deal not only with the event itself but also with his emotional reaction; this tends to overload the nervous system and cause excessive cortical activity, which increases the impact of the stimulus. He is therefore easily distracted and finds it hard to stay with one activity.

The left-brain-dominant person has trouble relaxing; his brain generates few alpha waves (low-frequency, "relaxation" waves) and much beta wave (high-frequency, "tension" waves) activity. Because of this, his waking and sleeping patterns may become disturbed.

The well-balanced brain has a natural ninety-minute cycle called the ultradian rhythm. During waking hours the brain primarily produces beta waves of alertness, but every ninety minutes it shifts into alpha-wave activity for a few minutes to allow rest and recuperation. The left-brain person, with his overproduction of beta waves, tends not to respect this natural rhythm and so gets overtired and edgy. This exacerbates his tendency toward insomnia, and he may resort to sedatives to ensure a good night's sleep. However, sedatives interfere with the dream cycle, which is the nighttime continuation of the ultradian rhythm. During sleep, the brain shifts every ninety minutes from its delta wave state (deep sleep) to a lighter sleep (paradoxical or REM sleep), allowing the occurrence of dreams to occur, which are essential to mental health. Sedatives tend to block this shift, resulting in deteriorating emotional health and further sleep disruptions. It is important for left-brain people to avoid this vicious cycle.

The individual with a dominant right brain has a concrete mind that relies on experience and a thought process based on intuition. He gives his projects careful consideration before carrying them out. He absorbs a great deal of information at once and integrates it gradually, a trait that allows him to consider highly complex matters. He has a calm mind, since his attention is focused not on a particular point but on the situation as a whole. His selective attention is wide, diffuse, and extensive.

On a neurophysiological level, his nervous system is calm and relaxed, as he has a great capacity for restraint. He quickly adapts to all types of situations and then takes his time assimilating them, thereby reducing the impact of a stimulus and allowing his body to absorb it gently. In this way his level of cortical activity stays low. He can relax easily and generates plentiful alpha waves. He tends to follow his body's natural rhythm in daily activity, respecting the ninety-minute rest cycle. His sleep is sound and restorative, and he tends not to rely on sedatives. Sometimes he is too calm and needs to be stimulated to become active.

Everyday Behavior and the Brain

Let us now turn to a detailed examination of the everyday behavior of left-brain and right-brain people.

The left brain is that of the thinker who relies on logic for the development of concepts. His mode of perception and activity is complex because he needs to analyze hypotheses in depth, testing out each step of his thinking. As a result, he is well suited to scientific undertakings. Because of his need for precision he attaches much importance to the meaning and written form of words (heir, air, err) and is precise in their usage. This helps him remember the words he has learned.

The left-brain-dominant person handles things one at a time. Faced with a sad or happy event, he is unable to place them in a more general context. His immediate reaction is strong; however, once the shock waves have passed, he will easily let go of this event and move on to the next. He does not dwell on the past and tends to be excited rather than depressed. The left brain is the brain of optimism, of positive thinking. It has been called the cheerful hemisphere.

The right brain is the mind of the artist. It rules the intuition, which presides over all forms of creation. It works through analogy and symbolism and can establish resemblances between objects that are essentially different in nature. As a result, the right-brain person can perceive, form, and create new images.[9] His thinking is based on concrete facts

---

9. In this context the word "image" is defined not as the exact reproduction of a person or a thing, but rather as the mental representation of a previous perception, feeling, or impression in the absence of the object that gave rise to it.

SUMMARY CHART

COGNITIVE AND NEUROPHYSIOLOGICAL CHARACTERISTICS OF AN INDIVIDUAL ACCORDING TO DOMINANCE OF LEFT OR RIGHT BRAIN

DOMINANT LEFT BRAIN	DOMINANT RIGHT BRAIN
COGNITIVE CHARACTERISTICS	
• Underinclusive	• Overinclusive
• Fragmented	• Complex
• Linear thought	• Circular thought
• Alert mind (beta waves)	• Calm mind (alpha waves)
• Intensive attention	• Extensive attention
• Selective, narrow, specific attention	• Inclusive, wide, diffuse attention
• Strong attention control	• Weak attention control
NEUROPHYSIOLOGICAL CHARACTERISTICS	
• Tense, agitated nervous system	• Relaxed, calm nervous system
• Weak reactive inhibition, slow to arrive and quick to dissipate	• Strong reactive inhibition, quick to arrive and slow to dissipate
• Brain waves in high modulation when awake	• Brain waves in low modulation when awake
• High cortical excitability	• Low cortical excitability
• Stimulus amplifier	• Stimulus reducer
• Less alpha frequency	• More alpha frequency

considered in an objective manner. His memory stores everything he experiences, and he is able to place individual events in a broad context. The right-brain individual has an immediate and approximate knowledge of the world around him and does not need to test this knowledge. Thus it can be said that his modes of perception and activity are simple.

This systemic approach to life enables the right-brain person to reduce the impact of events in the short term. In the long run, however, they will have profound effects. Since his brain stores specific experiences, he tends to dwell on the past; this, added to his lower level of cortical excitation, can lead to depression. The right brain is the brain of pessimism and negative thought. It has been called the sad hemisphere.

If the left brain is the master of words, the right brain is the master of sound. The right-brain person identifies sounds quickly and easily, instinctively assigning the true meaning to voice intonations and placing them in their proper context. He easily recognizes songs by melodies only, and enjoys humming.

BEHAVIORAL CHARACTERISTICS OF LEFT-BRAIN-DOMINANT AND RIGHT-BRAIN-DOMINANT PEOPLE

LEFT-BRAIN DOMINANT	RIGHT-BRAIN DOMINANT
SPEECH	
• Readily enters into conversation	• Finds conversation difficult; is awkward in his speech
• Takes the initiative in discussions	• Is reticent in discussion
• Has a rich, varied vocabulary	• Has a slight vocabulary
• Gives complete, detailed answers to questions	• Listens and answers in short, simple sentences; tends to use signs, gestures, or isolated words
• Becomes glib	• Becomes taciturn
• Moves from one topic to another	• Tends to stay with one topic
• More sensitive to strong voice intonations	• More sensitive to subtle voice intonations
• Repeats the words he has heard quickly and accurately	• Is often unable to hear and repeat words
• Easily grasps the meaning of words	• Has a poor understanding of the spoken language, since the meaning of many words escapes him
• Easily remembers the names of things without necessarily knowing their function	• Has trouble remembering the names of things but often knows what they do
INTONATIONS	
• Average voice and intonations	• Less varied intonations

23

LEFT-BRAIN DOMINANT	RIGHT-BRAIN DOMINANT
• Lively and expressive voice; animated speech	• Monotonous speech
• Deficient perception and comprehension of tone of voice and melodic flow of speech	• Accurate perception and comprehension of tone of voice and the melodic flow of speech
• Cannot easily distinguish between male and female voices	• Easily distinguishes between male and female voices
• Less attentive to words, as he easily recognizes their meaning	• Sustained attention to words in order to grasp their meaning
• More attentive to nonverbal sounds (interjections, sighs, etc.)	• Less attentive to nonverbal sounds

AUDITORY IMAGES

• Inability to recognize complex sounds	• Easily identifies complex sounds
• Defective perception of musical images	• Fast and accurate perception of musical images
• Trouble identifying popular tunes song's melody	• Quick identification of a
• Cannot remember songs	• Remembers songs easily
• Sings off-key	• Sings in tune
• Prefers to keep the beat without concern for the melody	• Prefers the melody to the beat
• Feels compelled to talk	• Feels compelled to hum

VISUAL IMAGES

• Good perception of visual images and everything concerning them	• Deficient perception of visual images
• Easily matches similar geometric figures	• Unable to match similar geometric figures
• No difficulty identifying incomplete drawings	• Difficulty identifying incomplete drawings
• Quickly finds the missing details in a drawing	• Unable to find the missing details in a drawing
• Groups numbers in terms of their visual aspect: V and X, 5 and 10	• Groups numbers in terms of abstract criteria: V and 5, X and 10

The Left and Right Hemispheres of the Brain

LEFT-BRAIN DOMINANT	RIGHT-BRAIN DOMINANT
MEMORY	
• Remembers theories learned in school	• Forgets most theories learned in school
• Memorizes recently learned words and remembers them for a long time	• Has trouble remembering words recently learned, generally forgetting them within two hours
• Good memory for verbal images	• Good memory for nonverbal images
• Unable to remember irregularly shaped figures	• Memorizes strange shapes and can identify them several hours after the initial experience
ORIENTATION	
• Good verbal orientation; ability to structure sentences well	• Appears completely disoriented verbally; sentences poorly structured
• Forgets to check environmental details, upsetting his spatial orientation	• Checks out everything; notices details and orients himself accordingly
• Moves too quickly and trips often	• Moves about easily
• Orients to external world	• Orients to internal world
EMOTIONAL TONE	
• Positive emotional tone	• Negative emotional tone
• Optimist	• Pessimist
• Cheerful, joyous	• Sad, morose
• Sociable, playful, easy to live with	• Closed in on himself, sullen, harder to live with
• Smiles; loves jokes	• Has trouble shedding his dark thoughts
• Interested in new things	• Not particularly interested in anything new
• Verbalizes feelings easily	• Keeps his feelings to himself
• Quick to become anxious, and also easily reassured	• Slow to get depressed, and also slow to come out of it
CAREER	
• Finds it easy to choose a career	• Has a hard time choosing a career

25

LEFT-BRAIN DOMINANT	RIGHT-BRAIN DOMINANT
• Facility for learning languages	• Facility for writing
• Studies the sciences	• Studies humanities
• Excels at mathematics	• Excels at music-making
• Intellectual	• Artistic

PHYSICAL HEALTH	
• Has difficulty relaxing	• Relaxes easily
• Higher muscle tone	• Lower muscle tone
• Generates more beta waves, fewer alpha waves	• Generates more alpha waves, fewer beta waves
• Sleeps less; tends toward insomnia	• Sleeps soundly
• Needs calming; enjoys cool colors	• Needs stimulating; enjoys warm colors
• Difficult to hypnotize	• Easy to hypnotize
• Tendency toward twitches, muscular spasms, headaches, acute and spasmodic illnesses	• Tendency toward asthma, depression, chronic and atonic illnesses

This mass of information may seem bewildering to you at first, but with some time and consideration it will begin to make sense. To help this process, I offer a final summary of the main features of the left and right hemispheres.

SUMMARY OF FUNCTIONS OF THE BRAIN HEMISPHERES

LEFT BRAIN	RIGHT BRAIN
• Thinker	• Artist
• Logical and abstract thought	• Concrete thought and formation of images
• Literal meaning of words	• Implied meaning of words
• Form of words	• Perception of content
• Uses concepts or theories in thought process	• Associates with experiences or objects in thought process
• Analytical perception	• Global perception
• Optimism	• Pessimism
• Verbal memory	• Memory of individual phenomena and objects

3

Identifying Your Dominant Hemisphere

The purpose of the following questionnaire[10] is to help you discover which of your brain hemispheres is the dominant one, so that you can correctly apply reflexology practices to free energies bound in the dominant brain and harmonize the body systems. I suggest you answer the questionnaire now, and then answer it again after you finish this chapter. To get the most accurate results, try to imagine you are experiencing the situations described in the questionnaire for the first time in your life. Record your immediate impulse, not your considered choice. There are no right or wrong answers. The questions serve only to help you determine your type.

Are You a Visual (Left-Brain) or an Auditory (Right-Brain) Person?

1. Someone talks to you in a loud voice. Does this

    A. Upset you and make you stop what you are doing?

    B. Leave you confused, wondering what the person's problem is?

---

10. This questionnaire, developed by Madeleine Turgeon, was inspired by those of Raymond Lafontaine and Ivon Robert. Lafontaine, *Etes-vous auditif ou visuel?*, pp. 7–8, and Robert, *La pédagogie des visuel-les et les auditif-ves*, pp. 49–51.

2. Someone speaks to you in a low voice. Does this

    A. Annoy you because it is such an effort to understand what is being said?

    B. Put you at ease, since it does not call attention to you?

3. Do you prefer to take a course where

    A. The teacher does most of the talking?

    B. The teacher encourages discussion with students?

4. Faced with a new piece of equipment, do you tend to

    A. Read the instructions before using it?

    B. Try to get it to work before reading the instructions?

5. When you have a problem, do you tend to seek

    A. Short-term solutions?

    B. Long-term solutions?

6. When you go somewhere for the first time, what first attracts your attention?

    A. The colors (of walls, furniture, carpets, etc.)

    B. The general look of the place (shape and size of rooms, furniture, etc.)

7. If you are expecting someone who arrives late

    A. Do you let it pass without saying anything?

    B. Do you say something at the first opportunity?

8. Faced with an unexpected setback (for instance, your car breaks down), do you tend to

    A. Feel disappointed, but deal with the situation?

    B. Become tense and edgy?

9. When confronted with a problem

    A. Do you consider various possible solutions before acting?

    B. Do you act before thinking things through?

10. When you are working, does sound

    A. Interfere with your concentration?

    B. Not disturb you much?

11. When people speak to you

    A. Do you want them to look at you?

B. Do you not particularly care whether they look at you?

12. Do you prefer to act

    A. Alone, asking for help only if you need it?

    B. With others, because of the mutual help?

13. Faced with the unknown, are you

    A. Mainly intrigued?

    B. Rather nervous?

14. When you watch television

    A. Do you comment aloud?

    B. Do you listen to the program, talking as little as possible?

15. To relax, do you prefer to

    A. Change activities?

    B. Sit and think?

16. When working on a project, what do you like to know first?

    A. The objectives of the project (the "whys").

    B. The way of carrying it out (the "hows").

17. If you hear a strange noise

    A. Will you go and see where it is coming from?

    B. Will you stay where you are and ignore it?

18. To get where you want to go

    A. Do you need a map?

    B. Are verbal directions sufficient?

19. In situations where you are meeting people for the first time, do you speak

    A. To one or two people in particular?

    B. A bit with everyone?

20. When you read a book

    A. Can you read long passages without losing concentration?

    B. Do you read a little at a time?

21. Faced with a decision

    A. Do you take the time to think the matter through?

    B. Do you decide as quickly as possible?

22. Do you tend to express your feelings

    A. To those you see regularly?

    B. Only to very close friends?

23. In the face of failure, do you tend to

    A. Feel solely responsible?

    B. Look for the causes of your failure within yourself and others?

24. What do you do with an empty cardboard food container?

    A. Break it and throw it in the trash.

    B. Keep it intact and use it as a waste container.

25. When you are assigned work, do you prefer to be given

    A. A detailed plan?

    B. General guidelines?

26. Do you prefer dealing

    A. With real-life situations?

    B. With hypothetical situations?

27. When you read, do you first pay attention to

    A. The meaning of what is written (the content)?

    B. The way it is written (the form)?

28. Faced with a new task, do you prefer

    A. A practical, "hands on" introduction?

    B. Absorbing the theory before moving on to the practice?

29. Do you prefer projects to be

    A. Long term?

    B. Short term?

30. When you ride a roller coaster, do you

    A. Scream or laugh nervously?

    B. Grit your teeth?

31. When people do not smile at you, do you wonder

    A. If they are mad at you?

    B. What their problem is?

32. Faced with a stressful situation, do you tend to

    A. Become tense and agitated?

    B. Become worried and slow down?

33. When someone raises his or her voice during a conversation, do you

    A. Keep quiet or change the subject?

    B. Also raise your voice?

34. Does a low, deep voice

    A. Not bother you?

    B. Annoy you after a while?

35. When you speak to someone and he or she does not look at you, do you tend to

    A. Stop talking?

    B. Keep on talking?

36. When you succeed at something, do you find that

    A. You do not seek out the approval of those around you?

    B. You love to be congratulated?

37. Is the way a table is set and food presented

    A. Very important to you?

    B. Not particularly important to you?

38. If you happen to displease someone

    A. Do you want to make peace as quickly as possible?

    B. Do you consider it not very important and feel that you can always make up later?

39. When you see a sign that says "Do Not Touch," do you find it

    A. Difficult to respect?

    B. Easy to respect?

40. When someone brings you food, what is your first reaction?

    A. "Oh, it looks so good!"

    B. "Oh, it smells so good!"

41. When you drive a car

    A. Do you look before backing up?

    B. Do you start backing up before looking?

42. In a car, do you buckle your seat belt

    A. Before starting up?

    B. The first chance you get after starting?

43. When you organize your drawers, do you

    A. Empty them out before sorting the items?

    B. Take items out one at a time, sorting them as you go?

44. When you drive a car, do you tend to

    A. Weave in and out of the traffic?

    B. Follow the flow of the other cars?

45. Do you

    A. Prefer eating meals at a regular time?

    B. Eat whenever you happen to be hungry?

To understand the results of this questionnaire, read the comments on the following pages.

A **visual** person would have responded to the questions with these answers:

1-A. He thinks that the person who raises his voice is angry with him. This prevents him from acting.

2-A. A visual person is annoyed when someone speaks to him in a low voice, as he must make an extra effort to hear.

3-B. Action makes the visual person think. He likes to exchange ideas with the teacher, as this helps him understand the subject matter better. He must comment immediately when a thought occurs to him, otherwise he may forget what he wanted to say.

4-B. As action helps his thinking, playing with the new piece of equipment triggers the thought process and helps him understand how it works.

5-A. Any problem worries the visual person. He likes to find solutions as quickly as possible, even if it means making a mistake and having to take corrective measures along the way.

6-A. The visual person's attention is drawn to everything around. He wants to see every detail.

7-B. The visual person gets agitated and worried when someone is late. He doesn't miss a chance to let the latecomer know how he feels.

8-B. A visual person is irritated by any event that upsets his schedule. His time is valuable and the unexpected glitch annoys him.

9-B. Since action generates thought, the visual person must act (speak, write, walk, etc.) to get his thought processes working on a solution.

10-A. An unexpected noise will shatter the visual's concentration, since it makes him lose his train of thought. He cannot easily pick up where he left off.

11-A. The visual person favors visual information and needs to have the speaker look at him.

12-B. The words and actions of others make the visual think and help him act. Consequently, he finds teamwork stimulating.

13-B. The unknown makes the visual person nervous. He reacts to the unknown with tension.

14-A. When watching television, the visual comments freely while still following the story.

15-A. The visual person can't stay with one task for too long—his attention is too concentrated. He needs to switch activities regularly in order to rest.

16-B. The linear mind of the visual person needs to know how the job is to be accomplished. He wants to know the procedure from A to Z.

17-A. The visual person favors visual information. Generally speaking, he will get up to investigate the source of the noise.

18-A. For the visual a picture is worth a thousand words and a map is worth a thousand explanations. You can bet that he will get lost along the way if he does not write down the directions.

19-B. The visual person wants to meet everyone. He feels that harmonious communication with others is essential for himself and all of humanity.

20-B. The visual person approaches reading with the same intensity he brings to other activities. His brain cannot withstand that level of concentration for long, and his mind soon begins to wander as one thought gives rise to another.

21-B. The visual person makes quick decisions and immediately goes into action. Acting as quickly as possible is a distinguishing characteristic of the left brain.

22-A. For the visual, expressing feelings is a way of releasing tension. As a result, he tends to speak of his problems to those around him.

23-A. The visual person feels fully responsible for his failure and wonders what he did to cause it.

24-B. Containers are important to the visual, and he dislikes destroying them. He prefers to reuse them wherever possible.

25-A. Because of his linear and sequential thinking, the visual person prefers detailed, preestablished programs.

26-A. A visual person prefers to deal with concrete situations. By trial and error he will come to abstract thinking.

27-B. The visual pays so much attention to the form of a text (grammar and vocabulary) that he sometimes forgets the content.

28-A. As the visual person learns to do by doing, he prefers to familiarize himself with a task by tackling it directly.

29-B. He is comfortable with short-term projects, as they allow him to quickly fulfill his potential.

30-A. He screams and laughs to release tension. Because he is unafraid to draw attention to himself, this is a marvelous outlet for the visual!

31-A. The visual person often feels responsible when faced with someone who doesn't smile at him, thinking, what did I do to him?

32-A. The visual becomes nervous in stressful situations, developing twitches that help release a little of the tension.

33-B. The visual speaks as loudly as others in a conversation in order to be heard. Talking is good for the visual person, allowing him to release tension.

34-B. Low, deep voices annoy the visual, since listening to them requires greater concentration.

35-A. The visual person stops talking when someone is not looking at him because he thinks no one is listening.

36-B. The visual tends to feel insecure and needs the congratulations of those around him to really savor his successes.

37-A. A nicely set table and beautifully presented food stimulate the taste buds and whet the appetite of the visual person.

38-A. The visual person absolutely has to please people. Failing to do so makes him anxious and worried. If he feels he has displeased someone, he will go out of his way to redeem himself.

39-A. The visual has trouble respecting a "Do Not Touch" sign. Since his hands are an extension of his eyes, touching something helps him understand it.

40-A. Since the visual relates to the universe through his eyes, he will exclaim, "Oh, it looks so good!"

41-B. Always in a hurry, the visual person tends to act before thinking. He starts to back up before checking to see if the road is clear.

42-B. The visual person will start the car before buckling up.

43-A. Since contents are of little importance to the visual person, he will dump the drawer out before replacing the items one at a time.

44-A. Traffic is always too slow for the visual. He tends to weave in and out of the traffic in order to get to his destination faster.

45-A. Live to eat! This is the attitude of the visual. Generally speaking, he prefers to eat at set times and finds it hard to skip a meal. His appetite increases when he gets upset.

An **auditory** person would have responded to the questions in the following manner:

1-B. The auditory person doesn't take it personally but does wonder why the person is speaking so loudly.

2-B. The auditory person is pleased when someone speaks to him in a low voice, since he is less likely to be noticed.

3-A. The auditory person prefers not to interrupt his teacher. He asks questions during the break or at the end of the class.

4-A. The auditory thinks before acting. He will read the instructions attentively before using a new piece of equipment.

5-B. For the auditory person, every problem deserves a solution, but not just any solution. He takes the time to think things out in order to find the most appropriate solution before acting.

6-B. For the auditory person, the most important element of a place is atmosphere, the overall feeling.

7-A. The auditory gets impatient when someone is late but tries to find a logical reason for the delay and waits to hear an explanation.

8-A. The auditory person is not unduly upset by unforeseen events. He immediately tries to come up with a suitable solution to the situation.

9-A. For the auditory person, thought leads to action.

10-B. A sudden noise will not disturb the auditory person too much, as his concentration is diffuse. He quickly picks up where he left off.

11-B. The auditory favors auditory information. He does not require people to look at him when speaking.

12-A. The words and motions of others often make the auditory person dizzy. He prefers to work alone, asking for help if he needs it.

13-A. The auditory does not lose his composure when faced with the unknown. He waits to see how the situation evolves.

14-B. The auditory person listens to the television. He refrains from making comments as this might prevent him from following the story.

15-B. The auditory stops his activities in order to relax. This allows him to reflect at leisure and sort out his thoughts before getting actively involved again.

16-A. The auditory's circular mind loves to know the objectives of a given project before beginning his work. If he considers the objectives to be valid, only then will he want to know how they can be attained.

17-B. If the noise does not seem threatening, the auditory person will ignore it. His ear easily tells him what kind of noise it is and where it is coming from.

18-B. Spoken directions are usually sufficient for the auditory to get to his destination, since his brain efficiently processes auditory information.

19-A. The auditory prefers to speak with one or two people rather than mingling with a whole crowd. Consequently, he will carry on long conversations and get to know new acquaintances in a more personal way. He strongly wishes to see humanity develop a better rapport with the environment.

20-A. When the auditory reads, his attention level is less intense than that of the visual reader. He can therefore read for longer periods of time without losing his concentration, since the rhythm of his brain waves is slower.

21-A. The auditory takes time to analyze every aspect of an issue before making a decision. The right brain thinks before acting.

22-B. Sharing feelings does not come easily to the auditory person. He rarely opens up, and then only with close friends.

23-B. The auditory does not necessarily assume full responsibility for his failure. He seeks to find the causes for it in others as well as in himself.

24-A. Contents are important to the auditory. He feels that the empty container has fulfilled its purpose and breaks it without a second thought, so that it will take up less space in the garbage.

25-B. Because of his circular reasoning, the auditory prefers a plan that can be modified to fit the circumstances. Fixed plans annoy him, as they prevent him from acting freely.

26-B. An auditory person prefers to reflect on hypothetical situations in order to plan future actions.

27-A. Content is of primary importance to the auditory. He excuses the author for a poor choice of words if he feels that the ideas expressed are valid.

28-B. The auditory never rushes into anything. He is confident about a task only when he has assimilated the theory behind it.

29-A. The auditory likes long-term projects because he can give himself to them more wholly.

30-B. The auditory grits his teeth through a roller coaster ride. Making noise would attract attention to himself and so would increase his tension.

31-B. When a person does not smile at him the auditory wonders, "what's his problem?" but does not tend to assume the blame for it.

32-B. Slowing down during a stressful situation allows the auditory time to think. He then becomes less anxious and is better able to assess the overall situation.

33-A. During a heated conversation the auditory person either keeps quiet to avoid a confrontation or changes the subject to create a diversion. He refrains from raising his voice.

34-A. The auditory enjoys people with low, deep voices; they do not draw attention to him.

35-B. The auditory person doesn't need to have the listener look at him in order to feel heard.

36-A. The auditory doesn't need the approval of others. He is capable of assessing his performance objectively and congratulating himself when warranted.

37-B. While the auditory person likes to see a beautifully set table, it won't make him hungry. But the smell of good food will!

38-B. The auditory likes to please, but if he fails he will not make an issue of it. He will simply wait for an opportunity to set things right.

39-B. The auditory has no trouble respecting a "Do Not Touch" sign. Looking without touching is fine with him. His mind quickly allows him to form an opinion of the things he sees.

40-B. The auditory person has a keen sense of smell. If someone brings him an attractive plate of food, he will first exclaim "Oh, it smells so good!"

41-A. Being naturally prudent, the auditory usually thinks before acting. He takes the time to look around before backing up.

42-A. The auditory buckles up his seat belt before starting the car.

43-B. Since contents are quite important to him, the auditory person removes items one at a time, sorting them out by category before returning them to the drawer.

44-B. Slow or fast, the auditory follows the flow of traffic

45-B. Eat to live! This could be the auditory's motto. If it were up to him, he would eat only when hungry. During trying times he loses his appetite.

You have just completed a questionnaire designed to help identify your dominant brain hemisphere. Don't be surprised if you found the results to be far from conclusive. To answer the questions you have to think about how you are and how you act; you must distinguish between your spontaneous reactions and your acquired behavior, which can be very tricky. To help you reach a more conclusive answer to this inquiry, I outline below six additional means for identifying your dominant brain hemisphere. In testing yourself, do your best to let your cortex—your intellectual mind—go, and let your nature—your reptilian brain—take over. The results of these tests combined with those of the questionnaire will likely reveal your dominant profile.

Eye Tests

The Direction of the Eyes

To find out if you are visual or auditory, arrange for a friend to ask you questions during the course of a casual conversation, so that you will be unaware that he is performing this test. He will watch to see if your eyes move to the left or to the right before you answer.

If you look first to the right, you are likely to be a visual person. If your eyes move constantly from right to left and left to right, you can be sure you are a visual. Only a visual person looks agitated for no apparent reason. According to the observations of Dr. P. Bakan,[11] the reason is probably that people with a dominant left hemisphere produce fewer alpha waves (the waves of relaxation). If, on the other hand, you first move your eyes to the left, you are likely to be an auditory. Your right brain is dominant and produces more alpha waves. The auditory person is calmer than the visual and moves his eyes more slowly and systematically.

Glancing at Printed Matter

Every week, flyers or catalogs are delivered to your home. Observe how you check through them. Visual people will tend to read from the first page to the last, directing their eyes first to the left page and then to the right. Their manner of looking will be the same with a newspaper or

---

11. P. Bakan, "The Eyes Have It." *Psychology Today* 11 (1971): 64–96.

magazine. An auditory person will generally start with the back page and move toward the front. Auditories focus first on the right page and then on the left.

Adding

It would be surprising if the visual and the auditory both added a column of figures in the same way. To illustrate their differences, we present seven three-digit numbers to be added.

$$
\begin{array}{r}
125 \\
648 \\
737 \\
546 \\
219 \\
334 \\
+\ 875 \\
\hline
\end{array}
$$

The visual generally adds the figures one after the other, his eyes moving gradually from the top to the bottom of the column. He proceeds the same way when he checks his answer, which he will do not because he doesn't trust the accuracy of his calculations but simply to make sure he was not unknowingly distracted.

The auditory glances at the figures to be added, looking for possible combinations (7 + 8 = 15, 9 + 6 = 15, 15 + 15 = 30) and he naturally adds them moving upward from the bottom of the column to the top. To check his answer, he looks for other combinations (5 + 5 = 10, 6 + 4 = 10, 10 + 10 = 20) and this time adds them working from top to bottom. Since he is not always certain of having mastered mathematics, he has been known to count on his fingers or with the tip of the pencil (discreetly, of course!).

Ear Tests

Humming

The visual does not have a particularly good voice. When asked to hum, he generally makes up a tune. If he chooses to hum a popular song, he will pick a simple one. No matter what he chooses, he often manages to sing off key or hum something entirely different than the song he has in mind. His performances are short and often end in a burst of laughter. (Better to laugh at yourself than have others laugh at you!)

It should come as no surprise that the auditory generally has a good voice. When asked to hum, he will think for a moment, select a song he knows well, and often hum it in its entirety without one off note. His ear is so good that he can easily imitate animal sounds and the voices of other people.

Ask: How Are You?

How do you respond to this general greeting? A visual person will be effusive in his response, answering "Fine, fine!" He will confirm it immediately by adding something to the effect of "I had a really lovely day. I did this and that. Everything went well. How about you?" To the same question the auditory will reply "Fine," and after a short pause will add "You?" He prefers to hear what the other has to say before expressing himself in his usual restrained manner.

In conversation, observe how you approach a question. When asked a direct question such as "What do you think of this?" or "I'd like your opinion on that," the visual person will talk a lot. The same question is likely to confuse the auditory, who prefers answering questions of a general nature such as "What's new today?" He will recap the events of the day in a manner that does not draw attention to himself.

Read Aloud

Read something out loud in a strong voice (without yelling), while alternately blocking and unblocking your ears. (An effective way of blocking the ears is to press on the tragus with the middle finger over the index finger. See figure 15, page 93, for identification of the tragus.) When his ears are blocked the auditory will read louder, faster, and with more self-assurance than when his ears are unblocked. The effect of reading aloud with his ears blocked is akin to an inner dialogue, so he is on familiar ground. The visual, on the other hand, is more comfortable reading when his ears are not blocked. Being an extrovert, his delivery is quicker and his voice stronger and more assured when he communicates with the outside world without interference.

Once you have conducted these tests and elicited spontaneous reactions, you should be able to determine your dominant hemisphere. Wait until you are fairly sure of your answer before using the reflexology techniques described in the following chapters. If you have correctly identified your dominant hemisphere you should feel an amelioration of your symptoms immediately following your reflexology treatment. If you don't feel the slightest change in your condition, or if you feel worse than you did before the treatment, check that you have properly applied the techniques. If you feel certain you have, then you can suspect that despite your best efforts, you have failed to identify your dominant hemisphere. In this case go back and apply the same techniques relative to the other hemisphere. It is important that the correct hemisphere be determined. Continued improper practice could produce negative effects.

Visuals and Auditories

It was in the 1960s that Dr. Raymond Lafontaine developed his theory of auditory and visual types. Through his clinical practice Dr. Lafontaine observed that the children he worked with interacted with the world in one of two distinct ways: one type seemed to interact primarily through the visual system and the other type interacted through the auditory system. As he followed these children through their maturation, he found that they stayed consistent in their ways of perceiving the world and processing information. From this observation he concluded that everyone could be classified as either auditory or visual. He spent the next thirty years refining and verifying his theory, which he calls Lafontaine's Principle. That is, regardless of sex, skin color, culture, or religious background, humanity can be divided into two groups: visuals and auditories.

When I first came across Lafontaine's Principle a few years ago I questioned, as you might, whether there was such a thing as an absolute rule that applies to everyone on the planet. I was also intrigued, as his categories of visual and auditory seemed to be very similar to the left-brain/right-brain distinction I was already familiar with. So I set out to test this sweeping assertion. Since then I have observed and studied my own behavior, the behavior of people around me, and that of people I meet during my many workshops on reflexology. The study grew into something of a game, and I became completely caught up in it. I analyzed everything in the light of Lafontaine's Principle. Like him, I finally came to the conclusion that everyone, without exception, is either a visual or an auditory.

I also observed that, as Dr. Lafontaine points out, all married or otherwise committed couples, harmonious or dysfunctional, tend to be composed of one auditory and one visual. This pattern seems to persist in the family that follows, in that children are born in visual/auditory pairs. That is, if the first child is an auditory, the second will be a visual, and vice versa. The third child may be either type, the fourth child will complement him, and so on.

The implication that each individual is *either* auditory *or* visual—not a combination of the two—may be difficult to accept. It likely contradicts your view of yourself or the apparent result of the questionnaire. To understand this problem we have to recognize that our instinctive reaction to any situation is so fleeting it often escapes our consciousness. Following this initial reaction of the dominant hemisphere we can and must move to the other hemisphere for a suitable and well-balanced response. The degree to which both hemispheres are open to giving forth and receiving information will determine how integrated and reasonable is our response. If communication flows easily between the hemispheres the response will be well balanced. On the other hand, a stressful state of mind or body will diminish communication between the hemispheres, causing us to become trapped in the dominant hemisphere from which we respond to life's challenges and changes in a way that may not be wholly beneficial.

The primary reaction almost always occurs in the same hemisphere and appears to be an innate mechanism that cannot be controlled by will or training. The secondary reaction appears to be much less spontaneous, and the ability of the nondominant hemisphere to participate in the response can be modified by training, reasoning, and willpower.

Almost everyone receives both auditory and visual answers to the preceding questionnaire. If you recognize yourself as one type in some situations and the other type in others, it is only because in one instance you reacted according to your typology, while in the other instance, although your immediate reaction was from the dominant hemisphere (according to type), your final decision or action was the product of a series of communications *between* the two hemispheres. This interaction may completely obscure the first, instinctive response, resulting in behavior different from that of your actual type. No one, it seems, is sufficiently aware of his or her primary reactions to obtain a 100 percent visual or 100 percent auditory score.

After a careful reading of this chapter the characteristics inherent to auditories and visuals will be more familiar to you. If you were to answer the same questionnaire at that point, it would likely yield very different results. Your new score would likely be closer to 100 percent visual or 100 percent auditory because of an increased understanding of instinctive response and heightened sensitivity to the initial messages from your brain. It is important to recognize that the primary reaction is neither better nor worse than the secondary one. It is the spark that lights the fire of cerebral activity. If we take the instinctive reaction and add to it the considered reaction of the other hemisphere, the resulting fire will be well fed, lively, and controlled (a sharp, quick mind), neither dying out from lack of fuel (depression, introversion) nor flaring destructively out of control (obsession, psychosis). If we can learn to modulate the shift from one hemisphere of the brain to the other, we will avoid many of the psychological ills prevalent in our society. When the brain is used wisely, health, joy, and harmony result.

The following chart[12] should help you better understand the psychological profiles of visuals and auditories.

PSYCHOLOGICAL CHARACTERISTICS OF VISUALS AND AUDITORIES

VISUAL	AUDITORY
COMMUNICATION	
• Attaches importance to the literal meaning of words.	• Attaches importance to the tone and volume of the voice as well as to facial expression.
• Regards the form as more important than the content.	• Feels the content to be more important than the form
• Gives detailed explanations.	• Gives short, succinct explanations.
• Prefers to amplify by plan or sketch, if possible.	• Does not require a sketch
• When he feels confident, he is extroverted and voluble.	• Generally quiet and introverted, he can, when feeling confident, talk a lot.

12. The profiles in this chart are based on material from the following books: Lafontaine, *Etes-vous auditif ou visuel?;* Meunier-Tardif, *Les auditifs et les visuels;* and Lafontaine and Lessoil, *L'Univers des auditifs et des visuels.*

Identifying Your Dominant Hemisphere

VISUAL	AUDITORY
• When he feels insecure, he tends to retire within himself.	• Taciturn, he gathers impressions and can suddenly explode, saying more than he intended.
• His face reveals his thoughts.	• His face is generally impassive.

CONFERENCES

• Needs a visual dimension, since theory and abstract demonstrations tend to distract him from what is being said.	• An excellent listener if the speaker is dynamic and the subject matter interesting. Focuses on the ideas rather than the words.
• Will remain at the conference even if he finds it boring, for fear of upsetting the speaker or missing out on something interesting.	• If he finds the topic boring, he will not hesitate to leave.

LISTENING

• Afraid of losing his train of thought, he tends to interrupt the speaker.	• Waits patiently for a speaker to finish his sentence. Can skip from one subject to another in conversation but remains focused on the main idea.

CONCENTRATION

• Concentrates so hard that he must rest frequently by switching to another activity.	• Has an ability for diffuse concentration, which can be maintained for long periods. He can carry out a task for several hours at a time without needing to do something else.
• Structures his thinking using reference points (sketch, chart, etc.).	• Organizes his thinking in a circular manner; digresses to resume his train of thought.

PERCEPTION

• Perceives components one at a time, adding them up to produce a whole (pyramid style).	• Perceives the whole and unravels its components like a spiral.

VISUAL	AUDITORY
ACTION	
• The master of action: he needs to move and act. He puts the cart before the horse, even if it means changing his course of action along the way.	• The master thinker: he goes into action after careful consideration and with all the necessary tools in hand.
THE NEED TO TOUCH	
• Needs to touch—touching is an extension of the eye. He must experience things and will touch the stove-top elements even if it means getting burned.	• Does not feel the need to touch. He will not touch the stove-top elements to find out if they are hot or cold—he will take someone's word for it.
HUGS	
• Gladly gives hugs but does not readily accept them	• Gracefully accepts hugs but is less inclined to give them
THE NEED TO PLEASE	
• Absolutely needs to please. If he thinks he has displeased, it is a disaster. He will do whatever he can to get back into the other person's good graces as soon as possible.	• Wishes to please. However, if he believes he has displeased, he will wait until a good opportunity arises to set things right.
• If someone around him looks glum, he feels responsible for the mood and wonders, "what did I do to him?" As a result, he often feels guilty when he's innocent.	• If someone around him appears to be in a bad mood, he will wonder what's wrong. However, he doesn't turn it into a personal issue, so he won't hesitate to establish contact.
THE OPINION OF OTHERS	
• Is highly sensitive to the opinion of other people. This makes him receptive to many ideas, but taken to the extreme it can cause him to constantly change his mind.	• Is not extremely sensitive to the opinion of others. Holds firm to his own ideas, sometimes to the point of stubbornness.

VISUAL	AUDITORY
WATCHING TELEVISION	
• Understands the action and the story even without sound. • Is not shy about expressing his thoughts during the program. He *watches* television.	• Can understand the action based on what he hears. • Misses out on part of the story if someone talks during the program. He *listens* to the television.
READING COMIC STRIPS	
• Understands by means of the picture, confirming it with the script.	• Understands by means of the script, confirming it with the picture.
PLAYING INDIVIDUAL SPORTS	
• Loves to practice individual sports but does not necessarily seek to compete. • Likes to practice sports with friends or family.	• Is quite comfortable with individual sports and prefers to practice them alone. • Loves to compete against himself, to test his own limits.
PLAYING TEAM SPORTS	
• Is not very comfortable with team sports. He plays mostly to win and to attract attention. His game is fast and centered in the moment; he is so focused on the action that he tends to lose his instinct for self-preservation and is likely to get injured. • If his team loses the game, he is deeply affected and tends to assume the blame. • To him, losing a game is not losing a battle, it's losing the war.	• Is comfortable with team sports. He plays for the fun of it. If he scores or plays well he will be pleased and proud, no matter what the outcome of the game. He is less likely to be injured because he remains aware of the dangers at all times. • If his team loses a game, he will accept defeat philosophically. • To him, losing a game is losing a battle, not the war.
DISCIPLINE	
• Is disciplined in terms of time. He likes to move within a well-structured framework and a set	• Is disciplined in terms of space. He needs to sort his things and file his papers so he can find

VISUAL	AUDITORY
time schedule. He is comfortable with routine but may be uneasy with the lack of imagination within it. He will satisfy this need by the way he does things, rather than upset his routine.	them easily. Whenever possible, he likes to operate within a flexible framework and time schedule.

SUCCESS

• Gauges his success by the reaction of others. • Needs approval, as he tends to underestimate himself. • Is comfortable with short-term projects because they allow him to quickly express his full potential.	• Gauges his success according to his own criteria. • Has relatively less need for outside approval. • May occasionally underestimate himself in comparison to the fast successes of the visual, since he does his best work on long-term projects.

FAILURE

• Gets upset about failing on the first try and even more upset if his failure is pointed out to him. He's not inclined to start over.	• Is always disappointed with failure, but will agree to start over.

REPRIMAND AND PUNISHMENT

• Rather than reprimand him, it is preferable to explain to him, as soon as possible, why what he has done is wrong and give the reasons for his punishment.	• Rarely caught with his hand in the cookie jar, he plans misdeeds and gets the visuals to carry them out. When caught, seems indifferent to reprimand.

PAIN

• Caught up in the action, he will not immediately notice pain. However, if he is bleeding or if someone around him appears concerned, it becomes a big deal. • He fears hospitals and has a strong need to be surrounded and reassured by everyone around him.	• Reacts immediately to pain and seeks help. If those around appear concerned, he will tend to reassure them, telling them there's nothing to worry about. • Dislikes hospitals, but will go if he feels it's necessary.

VISUAL	AUDITORY
CHANGE	
• Is enthusiastic about change and rushes into things without giving them much thought. Once the initial euphoria wears off, however, he starts seeking ways to handle his new state of affairs.	• Normally skeptical about change, he will observe and think before making a move. If he's convinced of the need for change, he will determine the best way to go about it before taking action.
ORDERS	
• Gets defensive when given an order. In dealing with him, it is preferable to express your needs as a wish or suggestion, which he will then gladly carry out. Even though he doesn't like taking orders, he will be the first to give them—very directly, at that—because he worries that he won't be properly understood otherwise.	• Waits for orders before acting and will carry them out in his own way. He will experience ambivalence in a "wish"; the ambivalence is likely to prevent him from acting.
TIME	
• Nothing happens fast enough—he has no time to waste. He operates in the present, feeling that to-morrow may be too late. He therefore tends to react impulsively to events, which can lead to problems. The visual wants to gain time now, even if it means losing time later.	• He will take the time to ponder a project and consider all aspects before carrying it out. Consequently, he may pass up excellent opportunities—his ship may leave before he decides to board. He is willing to take time now in order to save time later.

In all things, dominance of the visual or the auditory has a decided influence on our behavior. We have touched on some aspects of this in the preceding chart. A study of its different themes has led my associates and me to delve deeper into the subject and to make personal observations we would like to share with you. Some will make you laugh or smile as you recognize yourself in the ways of being or acting that we present.

Accidents

The visual can be said to "trip over the flowers in the carpet." In his rush to get what he wants, he fails to see the obstacles in his path. He will forget that the table is rectangular or that he is close to a staircase. His reflexes are quick, though, and will help him avoid head-on collisions or other serious accidents.

More reflective, the auditory takes in his surroundings with his eyes before heading toward his objective. If there is an obstacle in his path he will easily get around it, so there is no question of losing face by losing his balance. His hesitation may cause him to freeze on the spot and cause the "obstacles" (car, people, etc.) to run into him.

Automobile

Neither the visual nor the auditory person can be considered a "good" or a "bad" driver. Either can be exemplary or awful, obedient to or disrespectful of traffic regulations, but for different reasons. Let's follow them on a short jaunt from the time they get into the car until they park.

Who will be more likely to buckle his seat belt? Generally the visual will, but often only after he's started the car. (He thinks this will help him gain time.) If he considers the use of a seat belt to be justified, the auditory driver will buckle up before starting the car: he dislikes taking needless risks just to gain a few seconds. Before backing up he will look around and set his vehicle in motion only if the drive is clear. The visual will start to back up first, then check to see if he can safely do so.

On the road, both the visual and the auditory can get annoyed in slow-moving traffic—the visual because he is wasting time and the auditory because his cruising speed has been disrupted. The visual will dodge in and out of traffic to reach his destination quickly, whereas the auditory will accept the pace of the traffic even if it's not to his liking. At his destination, the auditory will take the first available parking space to be sure of getting one. The visual, on the other hand, will get as close to the entrance as he can, even if it means driving around in circles and losing a more distant parking spot that was available when he first arrived. In an effort to save time and be as close as possible to his destination, he will go so far as to park his car illegally if he thinks he won't be long inside.

50

Gifts

Do you want to make a visual person happy? Whatever you do, don't give him something practical or useful. He views these as necessities. The visual person likes decorative and original items, containers (jewelry boxes, candle holders, etc.) and cut glass. Select his gift with care and wrap it beautifully. He'll be thrilled.

When it's his turn to give, he likes to surprise and make the fun last. To this end, he might give several gifts, each wrapped differently, or a single gift that might be placed in a second, larger box. A visual father hid a $50 bill in a hockey puck placed in a huge box full of paper. Imagine his son's delight when he discovered the money!

The way to please an auditory person is to ask him what he wants and give it to him. Do not try to surprise him: you may regret it. Unlike the visual, the auditory likes getting practical things, and even then they must be selected according to his criteria. You will never go wrong if you give him money to get what *he* wants.

The auditory gives what he would like to receive: money and other practical items. If the recipient is another auditory, great! The gift will be sure to please. If intended for a visual, however, such a gift will be a disappointment. The auditory will usually give a single gift, preferably one chosen in the presence of the recipient or after discussion with him. It is the gift itself rather than the presentation that is important to the auditory. He wants to be sure that the gift is appropriate and suitable for the recipient.

Leisure

Obviously these two types prefer different leisure activities. The visual will spend time watching television, going to the movies, watching sunrises and sunsets, gazing at the stars, taking in the scenery, window-shopping, decorating the house, photographing, reading (he sees lots of images), visiting art galleries and museums, people-watching, playing with computers.

The auditory's leisure activities will include listening to the radio or attending a concert; reading (he hears the words); listening to conversations; playing a musical instrument; giving lectures or speaking; playing with his ham radio; delighting in the sound of the water, the birds, and the wind; programming a computer; finding a way to reuse wood, string, glass, nails, and other such materials; getting outdoors to play sports or games of skill.

Fashion

The visual person shows a distinct preference for brightly colored clothes. Fabrics are generally silky or shiny, and for special occasions the visual will add sequins and lamés. The visual favors florals and other prints, often selecting those that hide much of the fabric's background. He likes to attract attention. The visual's closet tends to overflow, since he will often purchase clothing on impulse even if it doesn't match the rest of his wardrobe. He rationalizes the purchase by saying he will find something to go with it.

Interestingly enough, the visual's hair often has little curl. Hair can reflect one's mode of thinking—in this case, linear. Visuals tend to wear their hair short. The visual woman likes her makeup to accent her best facial features, especially her eyes. She generally wears large jewelry. After all, what is the point of wearing jewelry if no one can see it?

The auditory selects clothes in pastel shades, often tone-on-tone and cut from semigloss or matte fabrics. The auditory also favors florals and other prints, though these must be small so as not to overwhelm the background of the fabric. The auditory personality does not want to draw attention through eccentricity and takes great care to ensure that the particulars (hair, makeup, clothes, jewelry, accessories) form a total look that is both discreet and harmonious.

The auditory's closet has few clothes and those it holds are well coordinated. When shopping, his initial impulse is to put off the purchase of an item of clothing if it doesn't match what he already owns; he's afraid he won't find the right item to complete the outfit. As a result, he misses out on some good buys.

The auditory's hair is usually wavy or curly, reflecting his circular thinking. The auditory woman favors long hair. Her makeup is discreet, and she attempts to soften or conceal what she considers to be her facial flaws. She wears delicate jewelry.

In a fashion show, you can recognize the visual model as the one with a radiant, toothy smile and an expressive face. Her body is more restrained, with somewhat stilted movements. The auditory model, on the other hand, does not always smile, and when she does, she barely shows her teeth. Her energy is dynamically expressed through her body. Her movements are smooth and flowing.

Food

The visual person tends to cut food into cubes and large strips that he places in groups on the serving platters. He loves to create visual effects through contrasting colors—for instance, he will place carrots next to cauliflower and cauliflower next to broccoli.

The auditory, on the other hand, cuts food into small pieces and thin, round slices, placing them in a circle on serving platters. His guests will admire his presentation for its harmony rather than its contrasts.

At mealtime the visual is first to the table. He's hungry; his taste buds have been awake for a while. He will select one item over another from the plate, fully enjoying the contrasting tastes and colors. Conversely, the auditory must often be coaxed to the dinner table. As he expends energy in a more diffuse manner, he doesn't feel very hungry, although once he smells and tastes the food, his appetite will awaken. The more he eats, the more he wants. Missing a meal is relatively easy for the auditory person but hard for the visual. The auditory can fast more easily.

Health Problems

Faced with health problems, the visual is more likely to take solid supplements (vitamin pills), while the auditory tends to favor liquid forms (tinctures, tonics, and teas). The visual never has enough and the auditory always has too much. The visual stocks up on supplements but stops taking them as soon as he begins to feel better. The auditory brings home small quantities of medicine, taking them religiously until he has recovered.

Professions

An individual's profession is not always an indication of whether a person is visual or auditory. Objectively speaking, however, some professions are better suited to one profile or the other.

These careers attract visuals: film producer, graphic designer, cameraman, commercial artist, makeup artist, editor, hairdresser, house painter, clothing designer, optometrist, set designer, computer expert, photographer, engineer, decorator, accountant, art dealer, notary public, reflexologist.

Auditories are drawn to the following careers: writer; manager; music producer; ear, nose, and throat specialist; musician; lawyer; piano tuner; psychologist; electronic equipment salesman; massage therapist; sound engineer; radio announcer; guidance counselor; planner; programmer.

Advertising

Seeing an advertisement promoting an interesting new product, visuals and auditories will again respond differently. The visual, full of good intentions and wishing to save time, thinks, "I'll buy it and try it out. That way, if I ever need it, I won't waste time getting it." He'll probably opt for the most expensive and sophisticated model, still thinking, "I'll have what I need when I need it." He is a born experimenter but often does not have the time to explore the full potential of the equipment he buys.

The prudent auditory says, "I'll wait a while. This product hasn't proved itself yet, and the manufacturer will probably improve on it." When he finally does decide to buy, he shies away from more sophisticated models, rationalizing that the more complicated it is, the more likely it is to break. If he comes across a sale of a product he uses, he will stock up to make sure he has some on hand for a long time to come. The auditory plans for the future.

Storage

The visual organizes things vertically. The mail will be in a pile, as will his clothes and just about everything else. He will stack what goes on top of the counter, the desk, or the table, and he does this neatly, since visuals are important to him. However, the interiors of his drawers are often left unorganized. Being in such a rush all the time, he tells himself that he will straighten things out later.

When a visual loses something he will look for it throughout the house and enlist everyone around to help. If he remains relatively calm, his mind will be set to thinking and he will be able to picture where he last saw the missing item.

The auditory person stores things horizontally. He spreads out his mail, his papers, and his files on his desk with the idea that he would rather wait until he has time to put everything where it belongs. Otherwise, he thinks, he will never be able to find anything! If he misplaces something, the auditory will stop and take the time to ask himself where he could have put it. After a few seconds, he is likely to remember its whereabouts.

Senses

Visuals and auditories both use their five senses to establish contact with the universe—they just do it in different ways. While the left brain analyzes, seeing things in a linear fashion, the right brain synthesizes, using a circular mode of understanding. This basic principle is confirmed when we study the manner in which visuals and auditories use their five senses.

SIGHT

The visual has acute central vision. He analyzes the details of his environment one by one until they constitute a whole. His attention is first drawn to colors. As a result, his retinal cone cells, which are the most sensitive to color, do most of the work in seeing.

Auditories' initial view of their environment is peripheral. The auditory will take a place in with a single look, quickly noting shadows and lights, surface relief and depth. He primarily uses his retinal rod cells in seeing.

HEARING

The auditory has a selective ear and analyzes sounds with precision. For him, the melodic line of a musical piece holds no secrets—he can faithfully reproduce it. His voice is on key. People say he has a good ear.

The visual doesn't analyze sounds. Rather, he allows himself to be penetrated by sounds and then simply decides whether he likes them or doesn't. At a concert or recital, he will attach little importance to minor flaws in execution, fully giving in to the feel of the music and its rhythm.

SMELL

The auditory has a sensitive nose that enables him to readily identify odors. He recognizes flowers from their fragrance and foods from their smell. He reacts quickly to any suspicious odor.

The visual processes odors the way he experiences sound: emotionally. What matters to him is whether they are pleasant or unpleasant.

Since identifying them requires some effort, he will tend to focus mostly on the feelings they generate. Whenever possible, he will delight in those he likes and avoid those that annoy him.

TASTE

The visual enjoys the five basic flavors (sour, bitter, sweet, pungent, and salty), identifying them easily. He does not have to think about it; his "computer" is programmed to recognize them. The auditory, on the other hand, does not immediately recognize each of the five basic tastes but is more interested in whether the food suits his preferences. For instance, he may like chicken but not when it's served the same way twice, in which case he will tend to pick at his food, claiming that he is not hungry.

TOUCH

The visual has a strong need to touch what he sees. He familiarizes himself with his surroundings through a tactile analysis of its details. Auditories, on the other hand, do not need to touch to feel comfortable with an environment. Their peripheral vision gives them a general feeling for their surroundings, and that is sufficient.

Sexuality

The magic surrounding a pair of lovers, young or old, is fascinating. They seem to communicate almost telepathically. Their love links them like a golden cord. To know how to charm someone you must understand that with the visual, human communication starts with the eye, while with the auditory, it begins with the ear. Seeing and listening condition most of our human relationships. Taking them into account will help you understand and communicate your love.

If you want to communicate your attraction to a visual person, give him fun notes and things he will enjoy looking at—a beautiful picture, a bouquet of flowers. Use his favorite language. (Consult the "vocabulary" theme.) It's worth it—you will see his tension and resistance dissipate before your very eyes. How comforting for him to think that you understand him so well!

If you are involved in a love relationship with a visual, don't forget that he is aroused by what he sees, and he must see what he loves. Give him time to look at you. When preparing for lovemaking, take your clothes off slowly, one piece at a time. He is quite sensitive to the expressions on your face, and to put him in a romantic mood you may have to do no more than give him a special smile. He likes to make love in soft light because he wants to see his partner.

To balance his brain waves, he will choose to sleep on the left side of the bed (when looking from the foot of the bed) so that his dominant left brain can come into contact with his partner's right brain. In this way, harmony is created.

If you give him a massage, use firm movements—he does not appreciate tickling. Firm pressure reduces the accumulation of lactic acid in his muscles and relaxes him.

Strangely enough, while the visual lover appreciates your seductive way of undressing and your nudity, he tends to disrobe quickly and is somewhat uncomfortable being naked. The weight of his clothes calms his nervous system. For this reason, being naked is physically disturbing.

An auditory person will be aroused by what he hears. While he may not notice your new outfit, he will be interested in hearing about your day and will talk about his. He relates more to sound than to images and is more focused on the inner logic of words than on facial expression. When he is not talking out loud, he is talking to himself.

When you love an auditory, you must enter his universe of sound using his vocabulary. He likes hearing you say you love him and he likes to hear it often. Make up sweet and romantic endearments for him.

The auditory does not need the lights on to make love. Whether in darkness or light, the auditory is sufficiently at ease with his body to remove his clothes slowly and gracefully. If you give him a massage, you could caress him at length using light pressure—he will never tell you to stop. He deeply appreciates the stimulating effect of long sweeping strokes and light touches.

The Temperature

If you are visual, chances are you seek warmth: hot soup, hot water, warm clothes, well-heated rooms, southern climates. Warmth seems to soothe and balance your nervous system.

If you are auditory, you love to cool off, choosing cold drinks, lukewarm food, light clothing, well-ventilated rooms. You find winter sports invigorating. Cold stimulates your body, encouraging tone and generating energy.

Vocabulary

People often have trouble understanding one another. In a difficult conversation, each feels the other does not listen or does not speak his language. This feeling contains a core of truth. We must not forget that visuals and auditories each use a particular vocabulary that strikes a responsive chord in his brain, though not necessarily in your own.

When you speak to a visual person, use terms that evoke visual rather than auditory images. This is the language that goes right to the heart of the visual. Word images allow him to feel that you are on the same wavelength. He relaxes and opens up, feeling understood.

Here are some things a visual might say to you:

- I see what you're saying.
- I'd like you to see my point of view.
- That looks funny to me.
- It's quite clear.
- I observed that . . .
- If I could show you what I mean . . .
- Do you want to watch TV?
- My heart skips a beat when you look at me.

If you would like to respond in a way he will understand, you could say something like this:

- I see what you're trying to say.
- I can visualize your project.
- It doesn't look right.
- Let me see what I can do for you.
- What color would you see for this room?
- Could you shed some light on this?
- We'll see who has the last laugh.
- Looking at you sets my heart on fire!

When speaking to an auditory you will note that he instinctively selects words that express sound in all its forms. These are phrases an auditory is likely to use:

- Listening to you, I think I hear a ring of truth.
- Tell me about your plans.

- That sounds right to me.
- I love hearing from you.
- I heard through the grapevine that . . .
- This place is buzzing with activity.
- The sound of your voice is very soothing.
- Let's discuss the matter.
- I prefer a quiet place.
- Let's listen to the music.

To enter his world of sound, you may want to respond with such statements as these:

- You seem to listen when I talk to you.
- The sound of your voice is delightful.
- Tell me about your plans.
- You have a musical voice.
- I feel like singing.
- A bell just went off in my head.
- I like the tone of this conversation.
- Come. Let's talk.

By using words that evoke appropriate visual or auditory images, you will capture the attention of the person you're dealing with. He will feel comfortable and closer to you, convinced that you understand him.

Traveling

The visual and the auditory each have their own approach to travel. The visual will be ready at the appointed time, give or take five minutes. He will bring more luggage rather than less, just to make sure he has everything. He likes spontaneity, so he does not overplan his itinerary. He will have no problem making it to his destination on time if someone gives him directions and draws a map, but if the instructions are verbal, there is no guarantee when he will arrive.

The auditory is ready half an hour ahead of time, just in case. He travels light, carrying no excess baggage. He plans his itinerary long ahead of time and is unlikely to change it once he is on his way. Verbal directions are often enough for him; he just draws a map in his head while the directions are being given.

59

Proverbs

Finally, here is a game of proverbs and sayings. Read through the list, asking yourself which were spoken by a visual and which by an auditory. You'll find the answers at the end of the game.

1. *You can't judge a book by its cover.*
    (Appearances are often deceptive.)

2. *Strangers can lie with no fear of being found out.*
    (There is safety in anonymity.)

3. *Sufficient unto the day is the evil thereof.*
    (Take care of today's problems today.)

4. *He who hesitates is lost.*
    (To succeed, you've got to take risks.)

5. *Look before you leap.*
    (Plan carefully before acting.)

6. *Don't count your chickens before they're hatched.*
    (Wait until the results are in before doing anything.)

7. *When in Rome, do as the Romans do.*
    (Customs are different in different places. Act according to where you are.)

8. *Sleep on it.*
    (Don't rush into anything.)

9. *To thine own self be true.*
    (Do what you have to do and ignore the critics).

10. *Pace yourself if you want to go the distance.*
    (Make haste slowly.)

11. *Take care of the pennies, and the pounds will take care of themselves.*
    (Attend to the details, and the overall plan will work out.)

12. *A rolling stone gathers no moss.*
    (You won't acheive anything by skipping from one endeavor to another.)

13. *Once bitten, twice shy.*
    (When you've been hurt, you become more cautious.)

14. *While the cat's away, the mice will play.*
    (When the teacher or the boss is out, students or staff relax.)

15. *When in doubt, don't.*
(When you're not sure, wait before you do anything.)

16. *There's many a slip 'twixt the cup and the lip.*
(A lot can happen from the time you plan something until it happens.)

17. *Out of sight, out of mind.*
(Absence destroys affection.)

18. *One swallow doesn't make a summer.*
(You can close your eyes to an isolated incident.)

19. *Strike while the iron is hot.*
(You've got to make the most of an opportunity.)

20. *Opportunity makes the thief.*
(Opportunity can lead us to do things we might not otherwise do.)

21. *Familiarity breeds contempt.*
(When one gets used to something, it no longer seems so interesting.)

22. *Everything comes to him who waits.*
(With time and patience, you eventually get what you want.)

23. *Charity begins at home.*
(You have to think of yourself first.)

24. *Nothing ventured, nothing gained.*
(You don't accomplish anything by being too cautious.)

25. *He who laughs last, laughs best.*
(Laugh at others and others will laugh at you when your fortunes change.)

ANSWERS

Visual:
3, 4, 7, 12, 14, 17, 18, 19, 20, 21, 23, 24.

Auditory:
1, 2, 5, 6, 8, 9, 10, 11, 13, 15, 16, 22, 25.

4

Balancing
the Hemispheres

Breathing is the key to activating the nondominant side of the brain. Before we move into a discussion of how and why this is so, let us first consciously experience the switching of hemispheres through an exploration of paradoxical images.

Observe the drawing in figure 5. Inhale and exhale deeply while focusing your eyes on the drawing.

What did you see? When you inhaled, your eyes took in the positive space occupied by the illustrated object. You registered the figure—in this case, the chalice. When you exhaled, your eyes were drawn to the negative space around the object, or the background, the white area surrounding the cup. If your breath/eye coordination is good, you saw the profile of a face on each side of the cup when you exhaled. Being analytical and detail oriented, the left brain is drawn to and insists on finding meaning in the black shapes. It completely ignores the white background, remaining fixated instead on the figures it is programmed to process. To be able to make sense of the continuous white spaces it needs to work together with the right brain, which is not trapped by details. The right brain can perceive the whole pattern, unlike the left brain which builds a whole out of component parts. When the right brain engages, the pattern of a visual field leaps out at you and remains engraved in your mind.

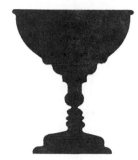

FIGURE 5: Paradoxical Image

Those of you who succeeded at this experiment showed that you could quickly establish contact between the hemispheres. If you had trouble seeing the different images, I suggest that you look at the drawing from a greater distance. If necessary, look at it from different angles or squint your eyes. Practice alternating between the hemispheres as you take in your visual field in daily life. Inhale and recognize the foreground, exhale and perceive the periphery, your entire visual field. Once your brain has discovered how to move from one hemisphere to the other in this type of activity, it will do so automatically.

Breathing and the Hemispheres

Just as proper breathing was essential to finding the face hidden in the paradoxical image, so is it the key that unlocks the door between the two brains, allowing one hemisphere to communicate with the other. Let us examine this vital activity in more detail.

Breathing moves the energy between the head, the pole of conscious awareness, and the pelvis, the pole of vital energy. When breathing, the body engages in a wavelike movement intimately linked to primitive life forms. Amoebae, fish, reptiles, and spermatozoa demonstrate the same basic movements. This primitive rhythm is at the heart of all life. It arises from the alternation of inhaling and exhaling.

The diaphragm is a thin, dome-shaped muscle that separates the thorax from the abdomen (figure 6). The diaphragm is constantly engaged during the breathing process; despite its thinness, this muscle is extremely powerful. It moves three inches down and three inches up with each breath cycle, executing roughly twenty-one thousand such

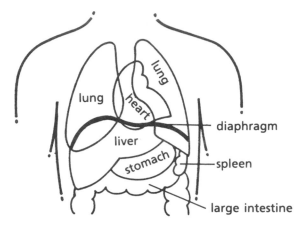

FIGURE 6: Anatomical Location of the Diaphragm

movements every twenty-four hours. As it moves, it compresses the abdominal blood vessels and lymphatic ducts, helping to propel the circulation of venous blood from the abdomen to the thorax.

During inhalation the diaphragm contracts, reducing its surface and lowering the top of its dome (figure 7). This increases the volume of air in the thoracic cavity and causes a swelling of the abdomen. The pelvis tilts slightly backward while the head tilts slightly forward, as if to get a whiff of a delicious soup.

The diaphragm remains passive during exhalation (figure 8). It is pushed upward by the abdominal muscular contraction, which also pushes the abdominal organs back and up, enabling the expulsion of residual air. The head then tilts slightly back to release the air upward. Humans exhale with their faces raised, just like the rest of the animal kingdom. Watch a bird sing, a wolf howl, or a cat meow. The expansion and contraction of the abdomen, and the consequent tilting backward and forward of the pelvis, involve the whole body in a gentle undulation.

Natural breathing involves the whole body, from the soles of the feet to the roots of the hair. During inhalation, the body's entire bone structure follows the movement of the rib cage, which opens and expands as the breath fills the body. During exhalation, the whole skeletal structure imitates the rib cage, which folds up like an accordion as the air leaves the body.

Full-body breathing is a practice we do not have to learn as much as remember. Infants and children who are lovingly raised maintain this

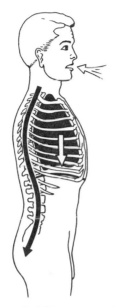
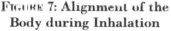
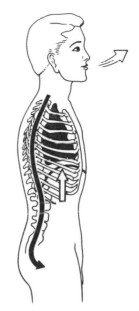

FIGURE 7: Alignment of the
Body during Inhalation

FIGURE 8: Alignment of the
Body during Exhalation

natural breathing pattern without conscious awareness. Indeed, full-body breathing fuels their abundant energy! Sometime, somehow, most of us lose touch with this ancient rhythm, and our breathing becomes shallow and incomplete. Stress and trauma will disrupt the natural breathing process, as will long periods of time spent in contracted postures such as hunching over a desk or leaning against a counter. However, this inborn capacity can easily be regained through awareness and practice. To help tune in to the fullness of your breath, you can breathe with your attention on any one of your joints. You should have the feeling that when you inhale the joint is inflating, and when you exhale it deflates.

The natural, wavelike movement inherent in the breathing process is vital to good health and imperative for free-flowing communication between the hemispheres of the brain. Practice breathing often: I recommend that you take three deep breaths at the start of any activity. You will be surprised to notice how much you inhibit your breath! With awareness alone you will find your full breath and the undulating movement that accompanies it. You can focus on, and gently exaggerate, the movements we have discussed, but never force anything or create any strain or discomfort. Your rhythm will emerge with gentle practice. This wavelike breath will energize and relax your whole body and open the pathways between the two hemispheres of your brain.

Other activities in addition to breathing can be employed to balance the complementary energies of the left and right hemispheres. An interesting perspective on harmony and relationship between pairs comes from traditional Chinese philosophy, which sees the world as an interaction of two basic qualities: yin and yang. Yin is associated with rest, receptivity, femininity, the moon, and inhalation; yang with action, aggression, masculinity, the sun, and exhalation. In the body, yin is in the feet, the front, the left side, and the right hemisphere; yang is in the head, the back, the right side, and the left hemisphere.

All disease is associated with an imbalance between yin and yang. Since the visual tends to have an overactive left hemisphere, he is likely to be very yang; he needs to calm his left brain and energize his right, yin hemisphere. Conversely the auditory, who has an overactive right hemisphere, tends to be very yin. The auditory needs to calm his right side and stimulate his yang, left hemisphere.

Visuals tend to overcharge the left hemisphere of the brain—the action side. Auditories overcharge the right brain—the reflective hemisphere. In this section I present four different categories—calming the left brain, energizing the left brain, calming the right brain, and energizing the right brain—and explain what activities will accomplish each goal. With this knowledge, you can balance your own hemispheres and ensure a more harmonious life.

Calming the Left Brain

Speaking out loud, using the hands for manual activities, and exercising or playing sports are yang activities controlled by the left brain. Such activities restore the visual person's energy balance. However, if he wants to endure without exhausting his energy, he must call upon his right brain, using the left side of his body as a point of support and balance when he goes into action. For instance, when he writes (a left-brain activity) with his right hand, he should rest his left wrist on the table. This helps him be more detached, and thus to be less absorbed in his activity. He will be less drained by it and more able to take breaks when he needs to. (Left-handed people see "For Left-handers Only" on page 69.)

During the course of a conversation, the visual must occasionally focus his eyes on a point to his left. This enables him to move between the form (left brain) to the content (right brain) with ease. Not only will he choose his words better, but also he will be in a position to express himself less emotionally.

When the visual holds an inner dialogue he overcharges his left brain, which is the speech center. The more words he uses, the more energy he accumulates—sometimes to the boiling point. A simple way for him to deal with this problem is to visualize himself either speaking to someone or in action. This will prevent the left brain from building too great a charge.

Planning a course of action has the same effect on the left hemisphere as the inner dialogue: it builds up energy. To prevent an overcharge, the visual must become an actor in his own drama—he must see himself carrying out each step of the planned action. For example, say you want to make a sandwich. To practice using the brain in the most balanced way, the visual should see himself opening the door to the refrigerator and taking out the bread, the cheese, the lettuce, the mustard, and so on, moving the activity through to completion in the mind's eye.

Energizing the Left Brain

The auditory naturally relies on the left side of his body (right brain) when executing an action. Therefore he must stimulate the energy in his left hemisphere in order to create balance between the two.

To move effectively into action, the auditory should bring awareness to the right side of his body. In conversation, he should look to the right from time to time. This will allow him to formulate his thoughts with greater accuracy and precision. When he writes he will notice that he automatically supports himself on his left hand, using considerable energy, while his right hand lacks energy. He should consciously focus attention on his right side. (The visual breaks the tips of his pencils, while the auditory does not press hard enough.)

It is to the auditory's advantage to conduct an inner dialogue. His left brain often suffers from lack of energy, and there is nothing quite like hearing himself speak internally to recharge the batteries. Another way for an auditory to charge his left hemisphere is to preplan every step of an action he wishes to undertake. The auditory should wonder to himself what kind of sandwich he wants, hear himself listing everything he needs, and then decide whether or not to make it.

Calming the Right Brain

Singing, drawing, and dancing are activities controlled by the right brain, and the auditory carries them out with considerable ease. They come naturally to him and help him relax.

The auditory usually sings on key, since the right hemisphere is the master of the melodic line. If he wants to enjoy the pleasure of singing for an extended period of time, he must call on his left brain (the hemisphere of mathematics and therefore of rhythm) by periodically looking to the right. This will help him blend melody and rhythm in a more harmonious way.

The auditory is particularly gifted in drawing, since he automatically leans his weight on his left arm (right hemisphere), which fosters creative thought. However, it is from the left hemisphere that we get the energy to translate our thoughts into action. For the auditory to draw for long periods of time without undue fatigue, he must occasionally shift his weight from his left to his right side.

The auditory moves through space with ease. His movements are undulating and fluid, and he is usually an excellent dancer. Still, if he wishes to avoid tiring too quickly, he must set his left brain in motion by occasionally looking to his right.

Just as the visual tends toward obsessive inner dialogue, the auditory person often gets songs stuck in his mind. Humming to himself compulsively can overcharge his right brain. If he wants to sing or otherwise engage that inner music, he should look to the right from time to time so his right hemisphere can operate without overloading.

Energizing the Right Brain

While the visual easily allows himself to be penetrated by the rhythm of a musical piece, he finds it difficult to sing or hum on key. He can call on his right brain for assistance by looking to the left from time to time. This makes it easier for him to carry a tune. When the visual hums to himself, he energizes the right hemisphere, which tends to need an extra boost. Humming to himself thus becomes a pleasant way of recharging his batteries. To sustain it for a time, he just has to look to his left occasionally.

The left hemisphere is the brain of flat geometric lines. To remember a panoramic view the visual must call on his right brain (the hemisphere of space) for depth. His right hand can give depth to his drawing only if he uses his left arm for support. This will help him to express himself more fully.

The visual person likes to be rocked by rhythm but does not always manage to express it easily. He overuses his right side, and this can throw him off. To dance to the beat, he simply has to look to the left occasionally and bring his attention to his left foot.

The left hemisphere controls the right side of the body, and the right hemisphere controls the left side. The visual uses his right (action) side to the detriment of his left side (point of support), while the auditory favors his left side over his right. The exercises I have suggested are designed to allow both the visual and the auditory to achieve a relatively good energy balance between the hemispheres.

Perfect balance would not be particularly desirable. Personal growth requires a certain level of tension between the two brains. If the imbalance should become too great, however, the excess tension could lead to a wide range of problems. Whenever you feel the physical, emotional, or mental tension that indicates you are locked in by your dominant hemisphere, use one of the methods proposed in this chapter. Don't let yourself be deceived by their apparent simplicity. In helping you restore contact between the hemispheres, they will allow you to carry out your activities with minimal effort and to live in greater harmony. What more could you ask for?

For Left-handers Only

From birth to four years of age, children sometimes use the right hand, sometimes the left, and sometimes both. Between the ages of four and eight years a preference for one hand over the other becomes definitive. Laterality—the use of one side of the body significantly more than the other—leads to undue fatigue and can even result in learning disabilities and speech problems. It is especially detrimental to left-handed people, who use the left side (the yin, or receiving, side) as a transmitter and the right side (the yang, or transmitting, side) as the receiver.

I was particularly interested in finding a solution to this problem, since I myself am left-handed. I pondered it at length and yet, when I finally did solve the problem, I was not even thinking about it. While having a meal, I realized that when I rested my weight on my left arm, I had no problem eating with my right hand.

It is important to realize that no matter what the action is, how you set it in motion is what counts. Left- as well as right-handed people must use their left hand for support and their right as a handling tool, thus respecting the laws governing brain and energy. There is nothing to prevent you from switching hands from time to time throughout the course of an activity, alternating your point of support. In fact, this is recommended, but only after *initiating* the action with the right hand.

The breath can be of great help in this process. The right side of the body is the yang side, and is thus associated with heaven. The usual process of initiating action is therefore to breathe in the yang energy from above, and, on the exhale, let this energy flow down the right side and into the action. On the other hand, when one wishes to relax he breathes in the yin energy of the earth, imagining that on the inhalation the breath comes up through the floor of the pelvis to fill the left side.

Left-handers, however, tend to reverse this coordination, breathing in through the pelvic diaphragm to initiate movement on the left. This disturbs the natural polarity of the body. To counter this tendency, the left-handed person should pay conscious attention, when initiating a movement, to breathing in the energy from above and exhaling down into the right side. This will help the right side to perform the action with skill. Once the action is begun, the left side will provide support for it. If a left-hander wants to wash a window, for instance, he should inhale deeply from above, then exhale into his right arm as he starts washing with his right hand, leaning some weight into his left arm to support the action. As he continues, he can switch arms from time to time.

This method can help eliminate fatigue, frustration, and even dyslexia! I have been using it for five years, and I now find it easy to use my right hand to do almost everything I did with my left. Many other people have enjoyed the same success. Try it for yourself and see how well your body responds.

5

Color and Sound
Reflexology

In the first chapters I explained the roles of the right and left hemispheres of the brain and helped you discover whether you fit the visual or auditory profile. Now I'd like to give you the means to apply this knowledge for better overall health and a richer, fuller life in which both sides of the brain are actively and expressively engaged.

In this chapter I will present my system of color and sound reflexology. This practice, when correctly applied, will free energies trapped in the dominant brain hemisphere, creating an unobstructed path for communication between the two hemispheres. This free flow of information balances the energy systems of the body and helps free it of pain. With this practice you can work directly upon the organs and glands associated with particular physical conditions, helping to stimulate the healing energies that bring the body to homeostasis. In a later chapter you will find a series of charts outlining the steps of this practice as it applies to a wide array of ailments. As explained in the introduction, I developed this approach through my research into both color breathing and Traditional Chinese Medicine, applying it to the theory of auditories and visuals.

Light and sound are forms of vibration; both can have a powerful influence on living beings. Some forms of healing involve the external application of specific colors and notes to affect the body. In this system we use sound and the image or the thought of color as internal touch to produce a healing effect.

Some of our ancestors in the healing arts, specifically the Chinese and the Hindu yogis, recognized the powerful effects of using sound and color for healing. They codified their practices, assisting us, many centuries later, in approaching similar practices with clarity. I would therefore like to introduce some of the theories underlying the practice of color and sound reflexology, in particular the Chinese Law of Five Elements and the Hindu chakra system.

The Five Elements

In the view of Traditional Chinese Medicine, the body's energy travels along a network of channels, or *meridians,* which serve to distribute and balance the energy among the various regions of the body. Each meridian is associated with an organ body as well as with a wide range of physiological and psychological functions. For example, the stomach meridian is associated not only with intake and absorption of food but also with digesting our experiences. Its organ-body association is the stomach.

In the Chinese philosophy all cyclical processes are seen as having five phases. These phases, or *elements,* are named "wood," "fire," "earth," "metal," and "water." Each element is associated with a wide range of phenomena, including colors, sounds, tastes, seasons, and the organs and meridians of the body. The table below shows these associations.

ASSOCIATIONS IN THE CHINESE LAW OF FIVE ELEMENTS					
Element	**Yang Organ**	**Yin Organ**	**Color**	**Note**	**Body Systems**
Wood	Gallbladder (GB)	Liver (Li)	Green	A	Muscular and lymphatic
Fire	Small intestine (SI)	Heart (Ht)	Red	C	Cardiovascular and reproductive
Earth	Stomach (St)	Spleen (Sp)	Yellow	F	Nervous and digestive
Metal	Colon (Co)	Lungs (Lu)	White	G	Respiratory
Water	Bladder (Bl)	Kidney (Ki)	Blue	D	Skeletal, urinary, and endocrine

The five elements interrelate as five stages of a cycle and are therefore represented around the circumference of a circle, with the yin-organ correspondence on the inside and the yang-organ correspondence on the outside (figure 9). The five elements principally interact in the generation cycle, indicated by the clockwise arrows linking the elements around the circle, and in the control cycle, shown by the arrows linking the elements across the circle. (It should here be pointed out that Chinese medicine is a complex system, interpretations of which differ among various schools of thought. Some of the attributions that I make may contradict other sources, but I have used these interpretations for many years with good results.)

In the generation cycle—the cycle of assistance—each element receives its energy from the preceding element.

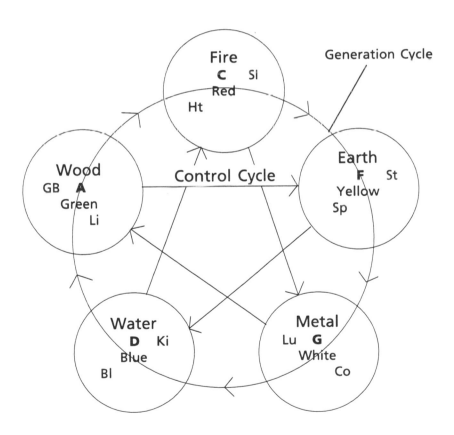

FIGURE 9: The Five-Element Wheel

- The wood feeds the fire. (Wood burns to create fire.)
- The fire feeds the earth. (Through combustion fire produces the organic matter needed to enrich the soil.)
- The earth feeds the metal. (The earth yields ores, which produce metals.)
- The metal feeds the water. (The minerals dissolve and enrich the water.)
- Water feeds the wood. (The water enables vegetation to grow.)

In the control cycle, each element is restrained or suppressed by another. The relationships between the five elements in the control cycle are shown by lines that form a five-pointed star.

- Wood controls the earth by holding back the soil with its roots.
- The earth controls water by containing it.
- Water controls fire by extinguishing it.
- Fire controls metal by melting it.
- Metal controls wood by splitting it.

Without the control cycle the generation cycle would produce tremendous overstimulation; the control cycle keeps the flow of energy even and balanced.

The visual—the extrovert personality—is associated with the yang elements of wood and fire, while the yin elements of metal and water are associated with the auditory—the introvert personality. Earth, the fifth element, serves as a liaison between the visual and the auditory. It is both yin and yang, representing the neutral energy of the center, the pivot around which the cyclical changes of the universe revolve.

The visual tends to overcharge the yang organs of the elements wood, fire, and earth (the gallbladder, small intestine, and stomach). The auditory overcharges the yin organs of the metal, water, and earth elements (lungs, kidneys, and spleen). In order to balance yin-yang energy we bring a yin color or sound into a yang organ and yang color or sound into a yin organ.

In this reflexology practice we consult the control cycle to harmonize overcharged elements. The colors and sounds employed are those associated with the element you want to affect according to your condition, as well as the color and sound of the element preceding it in the control

74

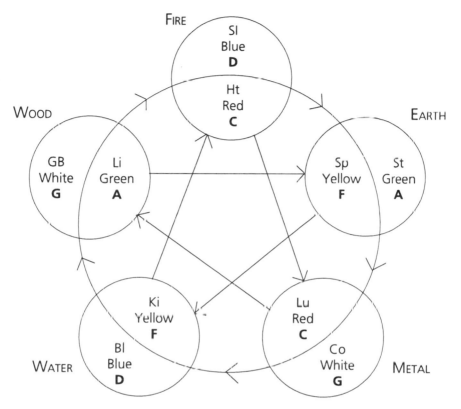

Wood: Muscular and lymphatic systems
Fire: Cardiovascular and reproductive systems

Earth: Nervous and digestive systems
Metal: Respiratory system
Water: Skeletal, urinary, and endocrine systems

FIGURE 10: Control-Cycle Relationships of the Five-Element Wheel

cycle. For example, the color for fire is red; the element preceding it in the control cycle is water, whose color is blue. Blue and red are therefore the colors we use to balance the fire element. Take a look at figure 10, which shows the five elements and their color and sound correspondences relative to the control cycle. Each circle in this illustration of the Five-Element Wheel shows two colors and two sounds. For instance, at the circle for the fire element you will see blue and the note D on the outside and red and the note C on the inside of the circle. When applying color reflexology to harmonize the meridians and organs of the body (see the third step, **Element**, throughout the systems charts), the visual will expel the color on the outside of the circle and breathe into the body the color on the inside of the circle. The auditory will do the reverse, first inviting into the body the color shown on the outside of the circle and then breathing out of the body the color shown on the inside of the circle. When applying sound reflexology, the auditory will expel the sound on the outside of the circle and breathe in the note shown on the inside. The visual will bring into the body the sound shown on the outside of the circle and then expel the sound on the inside of the circle.

Specific instructions on applying the control cycle to sound and color reflexology will follow the brief explanation of the Hindu chakra system and its relationship to the endocrine glands, another body system whose harmony is key to our overall well-being.

The Endocrine Glands and the Chakras

The endocrine glands are master controllers of the body's physiological processes. They secrete various hormones that powerfully influence the body and the mind. The seven endocrine glands are governed by energy centers known as chakras. Chakras act as transformers, bringing subtle energies down to physical levels and reducing the intensity of this energy so that we can absorb it and use it properly. Figure 11 shows the endocrine glands and their locations in the body.

Chakras store energy. If one of these energy centers is deficient it will impact on the chakra above or below. Each chakra operates at a slightly different frequency from those around it, and all accumulate energy in a slightly different manner. Chakras are also psychic organs— points of contact and interaction between the physical body and the more subtle energy body. Consequently, the energies born of our spiritual growth pass through the chakras on their way to transforming us at a cellular level. Figure 12 shows the locations of the chakras in the body and describes their associations with the endocrine glands, colors, and geometric shapes.

In cases of chronic illness there is often an imbalance in the chakras and hence within the endocrine system. This imbalance can be redressed by the simple technique of breathing the colors white and black (or the associated notes G and D) into the affected glands. The color white and the note G have a stimulating effect on all the glands, while the note D

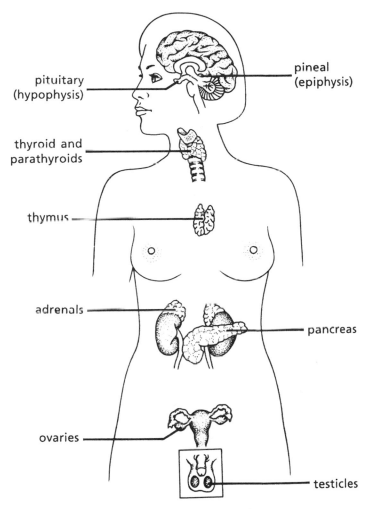

pituitary
(hypophysis)

pineal
(epiphysis)

thyroid and
parathyroids

thymus

adrenals

pancreas

ovaries

testicles

FIGURE 11: The Endocrine System

and the color black—which should be thought of as the soothing, velvety darkness of sleep—have a calming influence.

With this brief introduction to the theories underlying the practice of color and sound reflexology, we can now move on to instructions regarding its application. Following this overview of the system are separate sample practices for auditories and visuals relative to sound breathing or

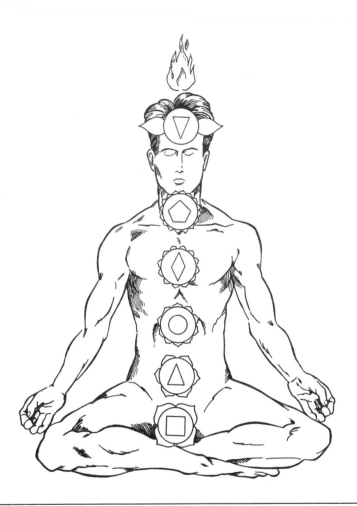

Chakra	Name	Location	Shape	Sound	Color	Corresponding Endocrine Glands
7th	Sahasrara—Crown	above and around head	Flame	B	Violet	Epyphysis
6th	Ajna—Third eye	center forehead, between eyebrows	Triangle pointed down	A	Indigo	Hypophysis
5th	Vishuddha—Throat	at base of throat	Pentangle	G	Blue	Thyroid and parathyroid
4th	Anahata—Heart	in heart area	Diamond	F	Green	Thymus
3rd	Manipura—Solar	in stomach area plexus	Circle	E	Yellow	Pancreas
2nd	Svadishthana—Sacral	in abdomen below navel	Triangle pointed up	D	Orange	Genitals
1st	Muladhara—Root or Base	base of spine	Square	C	Red	Adrenals

FIGURE 12: The Hindu Chakra System

78

color breathing. I suggest you read this overview first and then choose the appropriate sample practice to use in your first few sessions.

Practicing Color and Sound Reflexology

Color and sound reflexology techniques are powerful tools for self-healing. This system can also be used for the purpose of stimulating a healing response in others. In applying this system we first act directly on the affected area by breathing the sounds and colors associated with the earth element, the neutral energy between yin and yang. We then stimulate the glands associated with the physical condition we are trying to affect. The last step is to breathe the colors and sounds of the elements directly associated with the affected zone, using principles of the control cycle to bring the organs back into harmony.

The charts on pages 105 through 204 show the glands and the elements that are affected by various conditions of disease, directing you where to focus your attention when attempting to heal a specific disorder. Also listed are points on the ear to use in practicing auriculotherapy, or ear reflexology. This subject will be covered in detail in chapter six. One hundred seventy-four different conditions are addressed along with the colors and sounds employed to mobilize healing energies. The conditions are organized according to the body system affected. These categories are the skeletal system, the muscular system, the nervous system and the psyche, the endocrine system, the lymphatic system, the cardiovascular system, the respiratory system, the digestive system, the urinary system, the sensory organs, and the reproductive system. If, for instance, you have bursitis, which is an inflammation of the serous sac of a joint, and wish to use color and sound reflexology to help heal it, look up the condition under the category of skeletal system, as this is the body system in which bursitis appears. Similarly, if you suffer from asthma, consult the pages on the respiratory system for glands and elements to work with. Visuals and auditories will use the same colors and sounds for healing the same condition, with two significant differences:

- The visual will *breathe in* the same color or sound as the auditory *breathes out,* and he will *breathe out* the same color or sound as the auditory *breathes in.*

- Visuals will begin color breathing with an exhalation and

sound breathing with an inhalation; auditories will begin color breathing with an inhalation and sound breathing with an exhalation.

Once you have mastered color breathing if you are a visual and sound breathing if you are an auditory, I encourage you to try both approaches for an overall stimulation of your two brain hemispheres.

In preparation for employing color and sound reflexology, you should first envision the area that you wish to affect. Sit quietly for a moment, bringing your attention to this part of your body. Recognize that greater harmony and balance can be achieved.

Step One

You will begin your practice by working with the color or sound that controls the earth element: visuals will breathe out the color green or admit the note A; auditories will breathe in the color green or expel the note A. We begin each session by toning the earth element because it is the balancing element between yin and yang energies and as such it controls the functioning of the nervous system. Because of its pivotal role as the brain's messenger to the rest of the body, it is crucial to contact and begin to harmonize the nervous system directly at the place of dis-ease. Contacting the nervous system directly in this way will send a message of support to the brain and allow the nervous system to begin considering new expressions.

Step Two

After you have toned the nervous system in the area of dis-ease, you will move on to balancing the endocrine glands that are affected by your condition. The charts at the back of the book tell you which glands are relevant to your problem. We balance the glands by breathing black and white and the notes D and G. An even more powerful effect is gained by practicing the human crystal meditation, described below.

When you are breathing into and out of the glands, it is important to respect their order along the body's median line (consult figure 11). Where two or more glands are involved, when you expel a color or a sound you must first breathe it out of the lowermost endocrine gland and move it upward into the gland(s) above. Since a color or sound enters in a descending motion, the color or sound must be breathed in starting with the gland located at the top and move downward into the gland(s) below. This order must be respected at all times for the practice to yield beneficial results.

Breathing into and out of the glands is an effective healing technique. For those who wish to explore further, there is an exercise using the seven colors of the solar spectrum, all seven musical notes, and the seven geometric forms known as yantras. This practice is more complex and time-consuming; it is also very powerful and is therefore strongly recommended in cases of long-standing illness.

The practice of the human crystal is outlined below. The colors and sounds associated with each chakra respect Hindu tradition in every regard. The yantras, the geometric forms associated with each chakra, may be new to you.[13] I have described the practice in terms of color for the visual person and in terms of sound for the auditory; however, both can be practiced regardless of your dominant hemisphere.

The Human Crystal Practice—For the Visual

1. Inhale deeply. Exhale, seeing the breath glowing from the red square at the base of the spine outward into infinity.

2. Inhale, drawing the breath from infinity into the orange triangle at the navel center. Then exhale, letting the energy spread through the pelvis.

3. Inhale into the yellow circle at the solar plexus, then exhale toward infinity.

4. Inhale, drawing the breath from infinity to the green diamond at the heart center. Then exhale and allow the soothing energy to spread through the heart area.

5. Inhale into the blue pentangle at the throat center, then exhale toward infinity.

6. Inhale, drawing the breath from infinity toward the indigo triangle at the third eye; then exhale, and let the energy spread through the brain.

7. Finally, inhale and exhale through the violet flame at the crown chakra, radiating toward infinity in all directions.

---

13. Grateful acknowledgment is made to Madeleine-Andrée for the use of her yantra system.

When you use color reflexology in the human crystal practice, energies are constantly being sent out and taken in. Breathing becomes a golden thread that weaves out of the red square, into the orange triangle, out of the yellow circle, into the green diamond, out of the blue pentangle, into the indigo triangle, and out through the violet flame.

The Human Crystal Practice—For the Auditory

1. Inhale. Exhale, spiraling the note C out through the red square at the base of the spine. You needn't sing the note; it is enough to say "C" three times.
2. Inhale. Exhale, bringing the note D in through the orange triangle at the navel center.
3. Inhale. Exhale, sending the note E out through the yellow circle at the solar plexus.
4. Inhale. Exhale, bringing the note F in through the green diamond at the heart center.
5. Inhale. Exhale, sending the note G out through the blue pentangle at the throat center.
6. Inhale. Exhale, bringing the note A in through the indigo triangle at the third eye.
7. Inhale. Exhale the note B out through the violet flame at the crown of the head.

Step Three

The third and final step of this healing technique is to breathe the colors or sounds of the elements associated with the condition you are addressing. Having already acted on the nervous and glandular systems, we now act on the organs related to the problem. The systems charts in chapter seven tell you which elements and organs are associated with your condition. For many conditions there are multiple elements listed in step three. Because the interrelationship of our internal systems makes it challenging at times to determine which element is most strongly affecting the body's energetic balance, you should experiment to find the element that best responds to your efforts. Work initially with the first element listed in step three. If you feel positive results from your practice you can work solely with this element in successive sessions. If you do not feel results in your first session, work with the second element in your next sitting. By experimenting in this way and listening closely to your body's responses you will be able to determine which element is most influential in affecting your condition.

In order for you to correctly practice color and sound reflexology, I will now describe a sample practice for each of the four possible combinations of typology and technique: color breathing for the visual, sound breathing for the auditory, sound breathing for the visual, and color breathing for the auditory. Once you become familiar with the steps the actual practice is quite easy. However, there are different visualizations for the ways in which color and sound enter and leave the body, color having a linear energy and sound having a spiral energy. I suggest that you carefully read the instructions as outlined in the appropriate paragraphs below before your first few practices in order to apply the techniques correctly and thereby maximize the potential for bringing healing energies into your body.

Sample Practices

For the purpose of demonstration, let's say you are trying to heal chronic bursitis in your left shoulder. Turn to the systems charts in chapter seven; on the second page of the chapter you will find a listing of all of the body systems and health conditions covered in that chapter. Bursitis is an inflammation that occurs in the joints; it is therefore included in the section on the skeletal system. The listing on pages 100–104 provides easy reference to the section where you will find your condition addressed. In this case, the steps for applying color and sound reflexology to support the healing of bursitis are to be found on page 107. Turn to that page now and refer to the steps as outlined there while you read the following descriptions.

Color Breathing for Visuals

Before beginning your practice sit quietly for a few moments and direct your attention to the area of your body that you wish to affect. Relax your diaphragm and focus on the fullness of your breath as it travels through your whole body, including the area you desire to heal. Invite your being to come to balance.

When you are sufficiently relaxed, focus again on the specific area that needs healing, in this case the left shoulder joint, and begin step one by expelling from that area the color that controls the earth element. See the heading Colors in the systems chart; here it tells you that visuals should expel the color green from the area. As you inhale imagine the color ascending from within the shoulder area to the top of the shoulder joint. Shape the color into a ball. Now exhale and imagine this ball of color moving up and out of your shoulder area, and releasing into the atmosphere. Repeat twice more for a total of three cycles.

Next breathe in the color that benefits the earth element. Under the heading Colors you will find that visuals will breathe in the color yellow. Inhale, gathering the color yellow from the atmosphere. When you reach the top of the shoulder area, shape the color into a ball and let it hover there. On the exhale, slowly draw the ball of color into the shoulder joint. Repeat this process two more times for a total of three cycles.

Now we move on to step two, breathing color out of and into the glands associated with bursitis. From the systems chart you will see that these glands are the adrenals, the thymus, and the parathyroids; the chart also tells you that visuals will breathe out the color white. (For the location of the glands in the body refer to figure 11 on page 77). On a single inhalation gather this color first from the adrenals, then from the thymus, and last from the parathyroids, moving the color upward through the glands. Gather this color into a ball and then, on an exhale, release it into the atmosphere. Repeat two more times.

Now imagine the velvety, soothing black that you will breathe into the glands. On an inhale gather this color from the surrounding atmosphere and bring it down through the head and neck. Draw the color into a ball just above the parathyroids. On a single exhalation move the color downward as you "paint" first the parathyroids, then the thymus, and finally the adrenals with the color. Repeat twice more.

You're now ready to go to the third and final step of this practice. The listing at step three on the chart tells you that the element associated with bursitis is wood. In the Five-Element Wheel (figure 9, page 73) you'll see that the organs associated with the wood element are the gallbladder and the liver. On the systems chart note the abbreviations GB and Li shown next to the color to be expelled; these abbreviations tell you that it's these same organs, the gallbladder and the liver, that you'll be focusing on as you breathe. Because white is the color associated with metal, and metal precedes wood in the control cycle, white is one of the colors we use to balance the wood element. The other color employed is green, the color associated with the wood element in the generation cycle. Proceed with breathing as instructed for steps one and two, completing three cycles for expelling the color white from the gallbladder and finishing with three cycles for bringing the color green into the liver.

Finish with a few moments of quiet, letting yourself find the rhythm of full-body breathing. Then focus on the area in your body where your health condition manifests itself. You should feel a sense of lightness or increased energy in that area.

Sound Breathing for the Auditory

Sit quietly for a few moments and direct your attention to the area of your body that you wish to affect. (Again, we are focusing this practice session on the left shoulder joint.) Relax your diaphragm and focus on the fullness of your breath as it travels through your entire body, including the area you desire to heal. Invite your being to come to balance.

When you are sufficiently relaxed, focus again on the specific area of your body that needs healing, in this case the left shoulder joint, and begin step one by expelling from that area the sound that controls the earth element. See the heading Sounds on page 107; here you'll find that auditories should expel the note A from the area. Inhale gradually and imagine the sound vibrating along an ascending spiral that wraps *clockwise* around the shoulder joint. Then exhale, continuing to ascend the spiral, vibrating the sound *counterclockwise* along the spiral as it leaves the shoulder joint. Repeat twice more for a total of three cycles. (See

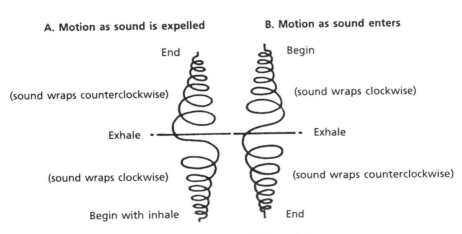

FIGURE 13: Sound Breathing

figure 13 for a representation of the course of the spiral during the inhalation and exhalation of sound breathing.)

Now breathe into your body the sound that benefits the earth element. Under the heading Sound you will see that auditories should breathe in the note F. Gathering the sound from the atmosphere, inhale gradually and imagine vibrating the note along a descending *clockwise* spiral. Position the vibration above the shoulder joint. Now exhale, vibrating the note along a descending spiral wrapping *counterclockwise* around the affected area. Repeat this cycle a total of three times.

It is important to note here that in working with sound, it is not necessary to sing the correct note—merely to sound the letter "A," "F," and so forth is sufficient. You can even practice silently by concentrating on the note. The right brain subconsciously knows the correct sound.

Now we move on to step two, breathing sound out of and into the glands associated with bursitis. As listed in the systems charts, these glands are the adrenal, the thymus, and the parathyroids. Auditories will breathe out the note G and breathe in the note D to benefit the glands. The instructions regarding the direction in which the sound travels are the same as in step one. On a single inhalation vibrate the note G *clockwise* along a spiral that originates just below the adrenals and ascends through the thymus and into the parathyroids. Then exhale, vibrating the note *counterclockwise* along the spiral as it ascends up and out of the body. Let the sound dissipate into the atmosphere. Repeat twice more for a total of three cycles.

Now gather the sound of the note D from the atmosphere. Inhale gradually and vibrate the note *clockwise* along a descending spiral until the vibration is hovering just above the parathyroids. Then exhale, vibrating the note *counterclockwise* as it descends through the parathyroids and the thyroid gland, coming to rest at the base of the adrenals. Repeat this cycle a total of three times.

You are now ready to go on to the third and final step. The systems chart tells you that the wood element is associated with bursitis and the sounds affecting this element are the notes G and A. In the Five-Element Wheel (see figure 9, page 73) you'll see that the organs associated with the wood element are the gallbladder and the liver. The abbreviations GB and Li next to the notes listed in step three indicate that these same organs, the gallbladder and the liver, will be the focus of your attention as you breathe. Proceed with sound breathing as instructed for steps one and two, completing three cycles for expelling the note G from the gallbladder and finishing with three cycles for bringing the note A into the liver.

Finish with a few moments of quiet, letting yourself find the rhythm of full-body breathing. Then focus your attention on the area in your body where your health condition manifests itself. You should feel a sense of lightness or increased energy in that area.

Sound Breathing for the Visual

The visual begins sound breathing by first breathing in a note to strengthen the sound energy that is lacking in his body. I will here describe the techniques of sound breathing for the visual, left brain-dominant person, again using the example of bursitis in the left shoulder joint as the condition we wish to affect.

In a mood of quiet, inward focus, direct your attention to the area of your body that needs healing. Relax your diaphragm and invite your breath to travel through your whole body. Recognize that your being seeks balance.

When you are sufficiently relaxed, move your focus to the place that needs healing, in this instance the left shoulder joint, and begin step one by bringing into that area the sound that controls the earth element. The heading Sounds on page 107 tells you that visuals breathe the note A into the area. Gather the sound from the atmosphere, then inhale gradually and imagine vibrating the note along a descending *clockwise* spiral. Position the vibration above the shoulder joint. Now exhale, vibrating the note along a descending spiral that wraps *counterclockwise* around the affected area. Repeat this cycle a total of three times.

Now you will breathe out of your body the sound associated with the earth element in the generation cycle; the chart directs visuals to breathe out the note F. As you slowly inhale, imagine this note vibrating along an ascending spiral that wraps *clockwise* around the shoulder joint. Then exhale, vibrating the sound *counterclockwise* along the ascending spiral until it leaves the shoulder joint. Repeat twice more for a total of three cycles. (See figure 13 for a representation of the spiral course of sound during the inhalation and exhalation.) Note that when you are working with sound it is not necessary to sing the correct note—merely to sound the letters "A," "F," and so forth is sufficient. The right brain subconsciously knows the correct sound.

In step two you will breathe sound into and out of the glands associated with bursitis. As listed in the systems charts, these glands are the adrenals, the thymus, and the parathyroids. Visuals will first breathe in the note G and then breathe out the note D to benefit the glands. The instructions regarding the direction in which the sound travels are the same as in step one.

Gather the sound of the note G from the atmosphere. Inhale gradually and vibrate the note *clockwise* along a descending spiral until the vibration hovers just above the parathyroids. Now exhale, vibrating the note *counterclockwise* as it descends through the parathyroids and the thyroid gland, coming to rest at the base of the adrenals. Repeat this cycle a total of three times.

To breathe sound out of the glands, on a single inhalation vibrate the note D *clockwise* along a spiral that originates just below the adrenals and ascends through the thymus and into the parathyroids. Now exhale, here vibrating the note *counterclockwise* along the spiral as it ascends up and out of the body. Let the sound dissipate into the atmosphere. Repeat twice more for a total of three cycles.

In the third and final step you will work with the sounds of the wood element, the element associated with bursitis. The organs associated with the wood element are the gallbladder and the liver (See figure 9, the Five-Element Wheel, page 73). The abbreviations GB and Li next to the notes listed in step three indicate that these are the organs you'll be focusing on as you breathe. Proceed with sound breathing as instructed for steps one and two, completing three cycles for admitting the note G into the gallbladder and finishing with three cycles for expelling the note A from the liver.

Finish with a few moments of quiet; let yourself find the rhythm of full-body breathing. Then focus your attention on the place in your body where your health condition manifests itself. You should feel a sense of lightness or increased energy in that area.

Color Breathing for the Auditory

Like the visual practicing sound breathing, the auditory begins color breathing with an inhalation rather than an exhalation. In the instructions that follow we will again be using the example of bursitis in the left shoulder as the health condition we desire to affect.

Sitting quietly, first direct your attention to the area that needs healing. Relax your diaphragm and focus on the fullness of your breath as it travels through your whole body. Invite your being to come to balance.

When you are sufficiently relaxed, focus again on the area that needs healing—in this case the left shoulder joint. Begin step one by bringing into that area the color that controls the earth element. The heading Colors in the systems chart directs auditories to breathe in the color green. Gather the color green from the atmosphere, and as you inhale bring it toward your shoulder. When you are just above the shoulder joint, shape the color into a ball and let it hover there. On the exhale, slowly draw the ball of color into the shoulder joint. Repeat this process two more times for a total of three cycles.

Now you will expel the color yellow from the area. This is the color for the earth element that is associated with the generation cycle. As you inhale imagine the color yellow ascending from within the shoulder area to the top of the shoulder joint. Shape the color into a ball. Now exhale and imagine this ball of color moving up and out of your shoulder area, and releasing into the atmosphere. Repeat twice more for a total of three cycles.

Step two involves breathing color into and out of the glands. As listed in the systems charts, the glands associated with bursitis are the adrenals, the thymus, and the parathyroids. Figure 11 on page 77 shows the locations of the glands in the body. From the chart you'll see that auditories will first bring the color white into the glands and then expel the color black. On an inhale gather a brilliant white from the surrounding atmosphere and bring it down through the head and neck. Draw the color into a ball just above the parathyroids. On a single exhalation move the color downward as you "paint" first the parathyroids, then the thymus, and finally the adrenals with the color. Repeat this cycle two more times.

Now imagine a deep, velvety black color. On a single inhalation gather this color first from the adrenals, then from the thymus, and last from the parathyroids, moving the color upward through the glands. Gather this color into a ball and then, on an exhale, release it into the atmosphere. Repeat this process two more times.

For the third and final step of the practice you'll bring into the body and then expel the colors associated with the wood element, the element most closely related to bursitis. On the Five-Element Wheel (figure 9, page 73) you'll see that the organs associated with the wood element are the gallbladder and the liver. The abbreviations GB and Li shown next to the colors in step three indicate that you'll be focusing on these organs as you breathe. Proceed with breathing as instructed in steps one and two, completing three cycles for bringing the color white into the gallbladder and finishing with expelling the color green from the liver.

Finish your session with a few moments of quiet. Find the rhythm of full-body breathing, then focus on the area in your body where your health condition manifests itself. You should feel a sense of lightness or increased energy in the area.

The powerful effects of this practice necessitate that you not perform more than six breath cycles for each of the three steps. It is also best to perform not more than three series of colors or sounds in any one sitting. For instance, if you've applied the technique to the area, the glands, and the organs associated with one of the proposed elements, wait until your next session to work on the organs associated with a different element. Finally, only practice *either* color *or* sound reflexology in one sitting. Do not immediately follow one practice with the other.

For acute conditions I recommend applying color or sound reflexology six times the first day, followed by three sessions a day for the next seven days. When healing a chronic condition apply color or sound reflexology one to three times a day for three weeks to three months. It will take this amount of time for the pain to dissipate. I recommend continuing with the practice for the same amount of time as it took the pain to disappear in order to rebuild the cells and fully heal the affected area.

Focused application of this practice will reveal its power. I hope you will find it beneficial in improving your health and that you will notice its effects in helping to unblock the energies lodged in your nondominant brain hemisphere.

6

Reflexology of the Ear

Another powerful self-help technique for balancing body energies is auriculotherapy, or reflexology of the ear, an ancient Chinese healing art that was revived in 1951 by Paul Nogier, a doctor from Lyons, France. Dr. Nogier conducted scientific investigations into auriculotherapy and thereby developed the first Western map identifying corresponding points between the ear and various areas of the body. Intent on making auriculotherapy accessible to everyone, two French physicians, Dr. Pierre Rosentiel-Heller and Dr. Maurice Amar, pursued the work Dr. Nogier had begun. Auriculotherapy continues to gain recognition and acceptance in the West, as it has proved to be effective in providing relief to people suffering from a variety of problems or ailments. I encourage readers to use auriculotherapy in conjunction with the internal practice of color and sound reflexology for the greatest results in self-healing.

Figure 14 shows a map of the ear based on the one developed by Drs. Nogier, Rosentiel-Heller, and Amar. The black dots show points on the outer surface of the ear, and the white dots show points on the inner surface. Points 19 and 26 are on both the exterior and interior surfaces.

The systems charts include the ear points that are indicated for treating various conditions. (The note ext. or int. at points 19 and 26 tells you whether to massage the exterior or interior surface of the ear.) To help you successfully massage the ear, I have illustrated its anatomy (figure 15). Refer to this drawing as you read the description giving the exact location of each of the points in the list that starts on page 92. The number for each point corresponds to the numbers in figure 14.

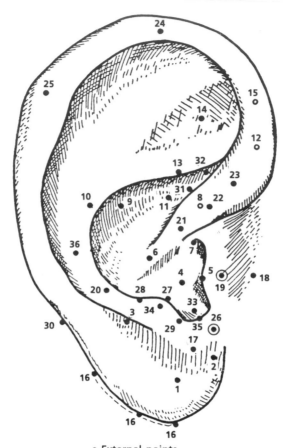

• External points
○ Internal points (points 8, 12, 15)
◉ External and Internal points (points 19 and 26)

FIGURE 14: Map of the External Ear

Ear Points and Body-System Correspondences

1. Eye: Master sensory point located at the center of the lobe. Reflex points for the pituitary and pineal glands are located in this area.

2. Nose: Nasal area reflex point, located at the center of the junction between the earlobe and the cheek.

3. Jawbone: Reflex zone located behind the antitragus, at the root of the fossa of the helix.

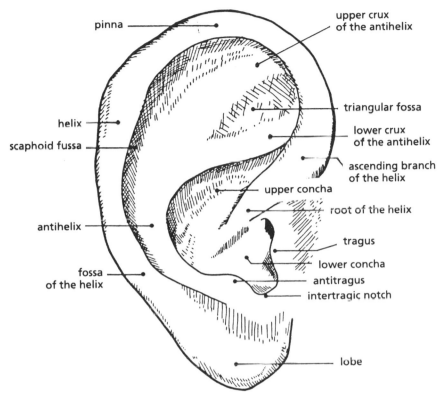

FIGURE 15: Anatomy of the External Ear

4. Lungs: Reflex point for the pulmonary area located at the center of the lower concha.

5. Ear: The zone affecting the auditory nerve is on the border separating the outer from the inner surface of the tragus.

6. Stomach: Reflex zone located at the very heart of the concha, at the base of the helix.

7. Throat: Reflex zone located in the upper concha, where the root of the helix meets the top part of the auditory meatus (ear canal).

8. Gonads: Reflex zone for the genital area is located behind the ascending branch of the helix, under the pinna. This point is related to the vagina, the uterus, the penis, and the prostate.

9. Spleen and pancreas: Reflex zone located in the upper concha.

10. Heart: Reflex zone located in the antihelix, at the level of the spleen–pancreas point.

11. Liver and gallbladder: Reflex zone located in the upper concha, beneath the antihelix.

12. Rectum: Reflex zone of the rectum and anus located at the tip of the lower crux of the antihelix, beneath the pinna.

13. Sciatic nerve: Reflex zone located beneath the triangular fossa.

14. Knee: Reflex zone located at the center of the triangular fossa.

15. Kidney: Reflex zone located on the axis of the triangular fossa, on the underside of the rim of the ear. (This zone is linear and extends from point 15 to point 25.)

16. Trigeminal nerve: Reflex zone located on the edge of the lobe. It innervates the chewing muscles as well as the muscles of the middle ear and palate.

17. Behavior: This is the master point for controlling aggressive or irritable behavior. It is also a secondary point for genital problems. It is located in the upper third of the lobe.

18. Master point of the tragus: This reflex point has an overall effect on the tonicity of the body, and is very good in treating fatique. It is also a secondary point for treating the external genital organs. It is located one inch in front of the tragal edge.

19. ext. Corpus callosum: This reflex zone strongly affects the communication between brain hemispheres and thus influences behavior and attitude. It also helps in the functioning of the autonomic nervous system, which controls such internal processes as digestion and sweat secretion. The zone is located in the middle of the tragus.

19. int. Skin: The internal aspect of this point assists with skin problems. It is located in the middle of the tragus on the inner side.

20. Shoulder: Reflex zone located slightly above the antitragus.

21. Point zero: Maintains the balance between the nervous and endocrine systems (figure 16). Reflex point located at the base of the ascending branch of the helix. This tiny zone is linked directly to most of the organs related to our vegetative life. Point zero can be used to eliminate hunger pangs in bulimics, reduce anxiety and nervousness, address weight problems (such as obesity or anorexia), or break addictions.

22. Lower limbs: Reflex point controlling sensitivity and movement in the legs, including the toes and soles of the feet. It is located just above point zero.

23. Upper limbs: Reflex point controlling the sensitivity of the arms. It is located slightly above point 22.

24. Allergies and sores: Reflex point controlling allergies and cold sores (herpes) located at the peak of the pinna.

25. Darwin's point: This point covers all cases of pain in the limbs. It is located on the thickest part of the edge of the helix.

26 ext. Anti-stress zone: Reflex zone located above the lobe and below the intertragic notch.

26 int. Point of synthesis: This point has an overall effect on mental functioning. Its internal location is just below the intertragic notch.

27. Posterior hypothalamus: Reflex zone located at the base of the antitragus, inside the concha.

28. Occipital point: This reflex point has an effect on sensory and motor problems of the limbs, joints, spine, and heart. It is located at the tip of the antitragus.

29. Genital point: This point affects the ovaries and testicles. It is located below the intertragic notch, in the top part of the lobe.

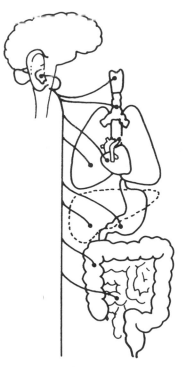

FIGURE 16: Point Zero (maintains balance between
nervous and endocrine systems)

30. Medullary zone: Reflex zone affecting the peripheral nervous system. It is located on the tail of the helix.

31. Intestines: Reflex zone located in the upper concha, near the ascending branch of the helix.

32. Metabolism and bladder: Reflex zone affecting metabolic problems. It is located at the center of the upper hemiconcha.

33. Anterior hypothalamus: Reflex zone located behind the antitragus, in the concha.

34. Sympathetic system: Reflex zone controlling the sympathetic nervous system is located in the antihelix.

35. Adrenal point: Anti-inflammatory reflex zone, located in the middle of the intertragic notch.

36. Thymus: Reflex zone located in the antihelix, between the zones governing the heart and the shoulder. Useful in the treatment of infections.

Figure 17 gives a visual representation of the point locations on the ear for the body's major joints and organs. This drawing will be helpful for memorizing general point locations.

Practicing Auriculotherapy

You can begin a reflexology self-treatment with auriculotherapy followed by color or sound breathing. Ear reflexology will directly influence the body systems, toning them in preparation for the more subtle influences of sound and color breathing.

An auriculotherapy session begins with massage of the dominant ear, the ear on which the indicated massage point is most painful. It is easy for a practitioner to apply simultaneous pressure (with the thumb and index finger) on both ears and determine, from the client's reaction, which ear is most sensitive to pain. Most people, however, are unable to make such a practiced determination, as they have little or no experience in this field.

Because auriculotherapy is so effective in relieving pain, I looked for another way of recognizing the dominant ear in order to make this practice accessible to as many people as possible. Here my knowledge of visual and auditory types proved most useful. Since the left (visual) brain controls the right side of the body and the right (auditory) brain controls the left side, it seemed that a visual person's dominant ear must be the right one and the auditory person's dominant ear the left. This theory was conclusively supported by my experiences with clients.

Having determined your hemispheric dominance, you next need to determine the exact location of the point you want to massage. To do so, hold your ear between your thumb and index finger and apply pressure to the specified zone. Move your touch around the zone until you feel a sharp pain. The pain indicates that you have found the exact massage point.

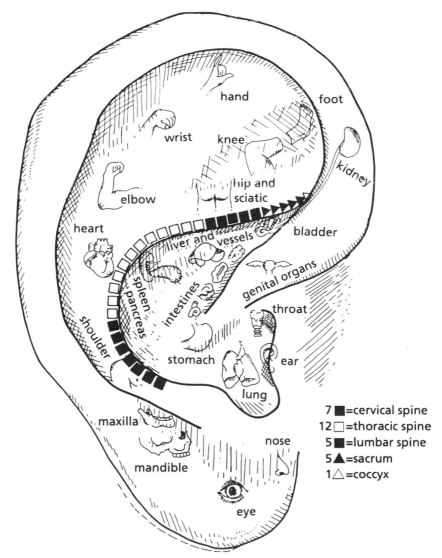

FIGURE 17: Point Locations on the Ear

97

Massage Technique

1. Begin with the dominant ear (right ear for the visual, left for the auditory), holding it between the thumb and the index finger.
2. Locate the points to be massaged by applying pressure and find the sensitive spots.
3. While exhaling, massage the point by applying pressure in a figure-eight movement. Stop massaging as you inhale, and relax.

Repeat the massage with this breath rhythm three times a day for acute conditions and three times a week for chronic cases. Because the energy is concentrated on a more superficial level and since energy travels faster on this level, acute health conditions respond to often-repeated treatments over the course of fewer days. Chronic conditions, on the other hand, result over time from deep-seated energy blockages and require less frequent massage over an extended period in order to unblock the energies and bring the body back to balance.

While there will be immediate internal benefits, your symptoms may not abate right away. As soon as you notice improvement, perform the technique once a day for acute conditions and once a week for chronic pain. Perform the technique two more times once the pain is entirely gone.

Do not massage more than three points in any one session. When more than three points have been associated to a condition, select the three most painful. The massage generates better results when performed from the reflex points of the head (lobe) working toward those of the feet (top of the pinna). In other words, begin your massage at the lowest point of the ear and work up toward the top. Make sure your massage is not overly vigorous; also take care that your nails are short enough to prevent injury to the ear. Avoid the use of probes or massaging instruments of any kind. These are designed for use only by auriculotherapy specialists.

The charts in the following chapter give you the ear points, sounds, and colors to employ in order to practice reflexology both externally (auriculotherapy) and internally (sound and color breathing). May these explorations bring good health to you.

7

Applying
Color and Sound
Reflexology:
The Systems Charts

The information in the following charts will guide you in your practice of color and sound reflexology. The charts delineate the colors and sounds to work with when you self-treat specific health conditions. Make sure to follow the three steps of this practice in their proper order; review the sample practices in chapter five (see pages 83–90) if you are uncertain about any part of the session. Note that for many conditions you are instructed to perform step one with your attention on the hypothalamus. The hypothalamus lies deep inside the brain; it receives all sense information originating in the peripheral sense organs, has an important relationship with the pituitary gland, and produces a variety of hormones affecting homeostasis. See figure 2, page 9, for a sense of its location in the brain.

Life-threatening or otherwise very serious conditions have been marked with "**Seek medical attention**." However, the persistence of *any* of these conditions, even those not marked, should induce you to consult a physician.

Paresis
Parkinson's disease
Sciatica
Stuttering
Trembling
Twitching
Vertigo

The Endocrine System p. 130
Allergies
Chills
Diabetes
Excessive thinness
Goiter
Hypoglycemia
Obesity
Premature aging
Stress

The Lymphatic System p. 136
Abscess
Adenoidal swelling
Cellulitis
Edema
Flu
Infection
Inflammation
Leukemia
Tonsillitis

The Cardiovascular System p. 142
Anemia
Aneurysm
Angina pectoris
Arteriosclerosis; Atheroma
Arrhythmia
Bradycardia
Cerebral hemorrhage
Coronary occlusion
High cholesterol
Hypertension
Hypotension
Myocardial infarction
Phlebitis

Raynaud's disease
Rheumatic fever
Tachycardia
Thrombosis
Varicose veins

The Respiratory System p. 152

Asthma
Bronchitis
Cold
Croup
Hay Fever
Laryngitis, pharyngitis
Nicotine-related ailments
Pleurisy
Pneumonia
Pulmonary emphysema
Rhinitis
Sinusitis
Voice loss

The Digestive System p. 160

Acid stomach
Aerophagia, aerocolia, intestinal bloating
Anal fistula
Appendicitis
Cirrhosis of the liver
Colic
Colitis
Constipation
Diarrhea
Diverticulitis
Flatulence
Gallstones
Gastralgia
Hemorrhoids
Hepatitis
Hernia
Indigestion
Jaundice
Nausea
Ulcer
Vomiting

The Urinary System p. 172
Cystitis
Enuresis, incontinence
Kidney stones
Nephritis
Renal insufficiency
Uremia

The Sensory Organs p. 176
THE MOUTH AND NOSE p. 176
Cold sore
Halitosis
Loss of taste and smell
Mumps
Nosebleed
Nose polyp
Pyorrhea
Stomatitis
Toothache

THE EYES p. 180
Atrophy of the optic nerve
Cataract
Chalazion
Conjunctivitis
Detached retina
Eye fatigue
Glaucoma
Iritis
Ophthalmic shingles
Sty

THE EARS p. 185
Buzzing in the ears
Deafness
Motion sickness
Otalgia
Otitis

THE SKIN p. 188
Acne
Burns, sunburns, cuts, stings
Dry skin
Eczema
Excessive perspiration

The Skeletal System

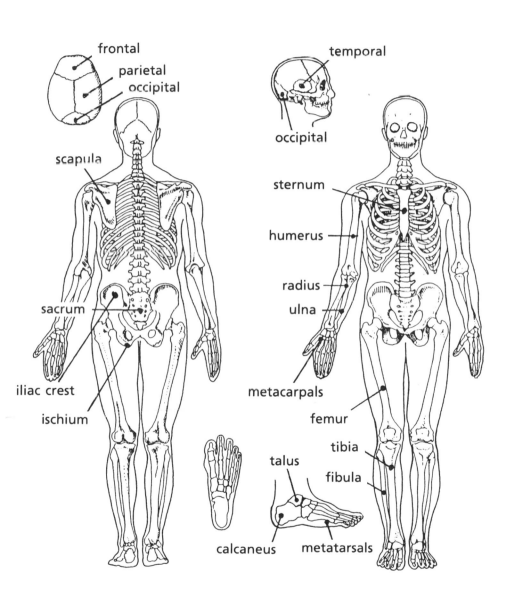

frontal

parietal

occipital

temporal

occipital

scapula

sternum

humerus

radius

ulna

sacrum

metacarpals

iliac crest

ischium

femur

talus

tibia

fibula

calcaneus

metatarsals

Ankylosis

Seek medical attention

Reduction or loss of movement in a joint as a result of abnormal joint-fusion.

Ear points: Affected area and 26 int., 19 ext., 30.

STEPS	COLORS		SOUNDS	
	V-Out **A-In**	**In** **Out**	**A-Out** **V-In**	**In** **Out**
Area affected area	Green	Yellow	A	F
Glands adrenals pituitary	White	Black	G	D
Element water	Blue (Bl)	Yellow (Ki)	D (Bl)	F (Ki)

Arthritis, osteoarthritis, rheumatism

Inflammation of the joints, tendons, or muscles.

Ear points: Affected area and 1, 28, 25, 21, 11, 31, 15.

STEPS	COLORS		SOUNDS	
	V-Out **A-In**	**In** **Out**	**A-Out** **V-In**	**In** **Out**
Area affected area	Green	Yellow	A	F
Glands entire endo- crine system	White	Black	G	D
Elements wood	White (GB)	Green (Li)	G (GB)	A (Li)
metal	White (Co)	Red (Lu)	G (Co)	C (Lu)
water	Blue (Bl)	Yellow (Ki)	D (Bl)	F (Ki)

Bunion (hallux valgus)

Swelling, often painful, at the bursa of the first joint of the big toe, sometimes accompanied by deviation of the toe.

Ear points: 9, 11. Also massage the area of the big toe shown in figure 17, page 97.

STEPS	COLORS		SOUNDS	
	V-Out **A-In**	**In** **Out**	**A-Out** **V-In**	**In** **Out**
Area big toe	Green	Yellow	A	F
Gland pancreas	White	Black	G	D
Element wood	White (GB)	Green (Li)	G (GB)	A (Li)

Bursitis

Inflammation of a serous sac, especially of the knee, elbow, or shoulder.
Ear points: Affected area and 35, 28.

STEPS	COLORS		SOUNDS	
	V-Out **A-In**	**In** **Out**	**A-Out** **V-In**	**In** **Out**
Area affected area	Green	Yellow	A	F
Glands adrenals thymus parathyroids	White	Black	G	D
Element wood	White (GB)	Green (Li)	G (GB)	A (Li)

Epicondylitis

Inflammation along the projection at the lower end of the humerus.
Ear points: Affected area and 3, 28, 23.

STEPS	COLORS		SOUNDS	
	V-Out A-In	In Out	A-Out V-In	In Out
Area humerus	Green	Yellow	A	F
Glands adrenals	White	Black	G	D
Elements fire	Blue (SI)	Red (Ht)	D (SI)	C (Ht)
metal	White (Co)	Red (Lu)	D (Co)	C (Lu)
water	Blue (Bl)	Yellow (Ki)	D (Bl)	F (Ki)

Fracture

Seek medical attention

Break or rupture of a bone.
Ear points: Affected area and 26 int. and ext., 25.

STEPS	COLORS		SOUNDS	
	V-Out A-In	In Out	A-Out V-In	In Out
Area affected area	Green	Yellow	A	F
Glands parathyroids	White	Black	G	D
Element water	Blue (Bl)	Yellow (Ki)	D (Bl)	F (Ki)

Gout

Painful inflammation and deposits of uric acid crystals around the joints.
Ear points: Affected area and 26 int. and ext., 28, 21, 17, 11, 15, 25.

Steps	Colors		Sounds	
	V-Out A-In	In Out	A-Out V-In	In Out
Area affected joint	Green	Yellow	A	F
Glands pancreas adrenals	White	Black	G	D
Elements water	Blue (Bl)	Yellow (Ki)	D (Bl)	F (Ki)
wood	White (GB)	Green (Li)	G (GB)	A (Li)

Herniated disc

Seek medical attention

Protrusion of the nucleus of an intervertebral disc, causing pressure on a
 nerve near the spinal cord.
Ear points: Affected area and 21, 22.

Steps	Colors		Sounds	
	V-Out A-In	In Out	A-Out V-In	In Out
Area affected area	Green	Yellow	A	F
Gland pituitary	White	Black	G	D
Element water	Blue (Bl)	Yellow (Ki)	D (Bl)	F (Ki)

Knee meniscus injury

Seek medical attention

Injury to the fibrous cartilage located between the two surfaces of the knee joint. May require surgery.

Ear points: 26 int. and ext., 22, 14.

STEPS	COLORS		SOUNDS	
	V-Out **A-In**	**In** **Out**	**A-Out** **V-In**	**In** **Out**
Area knee	Green	Yellow	A	F
Glands adrenals thymus	White	Black	G	D
Elements water wood	Blue (Bl) White (GB)	Yellow (Ki) Green (Li)	D (Bl) G (GB)	F (Ki) A (Li)

Osteoporosis

Seek medical attention

Decalcification of the bones, which become porous.

Ear points: Affected area and 29, 35, 32.

STEPS	COLORS		SOUNDS	
	V-Out **A-In**	**In** **Out**	**A-Out** **V-In**	**In** **Out**
Area affected area	Green	Yellow	A	F
Glands gonads adrenals parathyroids	White	Black	G	D
Element water	Blue (Bl)	Yellow (Ki)	D (Bl)	F (Ki)

Scoliosis

Seek medical attention

Lateral curvature of the spine.
Ear points: Affected area and 11, 15.

STEPS	COLORS		SOUNDS	
	V-Out **A-In**	**In** **Out**	**A-Out** **V-In**	**In** **Out**
Area spine	Green	Yellow	A	F
Glands gonads thyroid pituitary	White	Black	G	D
Elements water wood	Blue (Bl) White (GB)	Yellow (Ki) Green (Li)	D (Bl) G (GB)	F (Ki) A (Li)

Sprain

Tearing of the joint ligaments.
Ear points: Affected area and 26 int., 19 int., 21 .

STEPS	COLORS		SOUNDS	
	V-Out **A-In**	**In** **Out**	**A-Out** **V-In**	**In** **Out**
Area affected area	Green	Yellow	A	F
Glands adrenals pituitary	White	Black	G	D
Element wood	White (GB)	Green (Li)	G (GB)	A (Li)

Tendinitis

Inflammation of a tendon.
Ear points: Affected area and 35, 22, 23, 25.

STEPS	COLORS		SOUNDS	
	V-Out **A-In**	**In** **Out**	**A-Out** **V-In**	**In** **Out**
Area affected area	Green	Yellow	A	F
Glands adrenals thymus	White	Black	G	D
Element wood	White (GB)	Green (Li)	G (GB)	A (Li)

The Muscular System

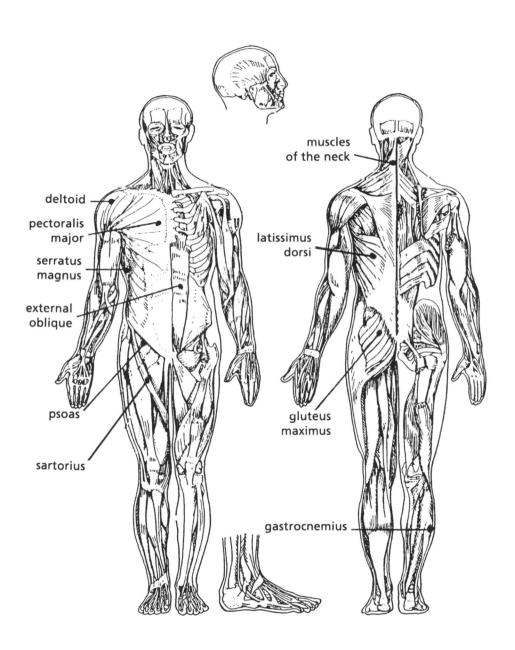

deltoid

pectoralis major

serratus magnus

external oblique

psoas

sartorius

muscles of the neck

latissimus dorsi

gluteus maximus

gastrocnemius

Cramp

Painful involuntary contraction of a muscle or group of muscles.
Ear points: 28, 19, 21, 22.

STEPS	COLORS		SOUNDS	
	V-Out **A-In**	**In** **Out**	**A-Out** **V-In**	**In** **Out**
Area affected area	Green	Yellow	A	F
Glands adrenals parathyroids	White	Black	G	D
Element water	Blue (Bl)	Yellow (Ki)	D (Bl)	F (Ki)

Myasthenia

Seek medical attention

Muscle weakness without atrophy.
Ear points: 35, 34, 21, 11.

STEPS	COLORS		SOUNDS	
	V-Out **A-In**	**In** **Out**	**A-Out** **V-In**	**In** **Out**
Area entire muscu- lar system	Green	Yellow	A	F
Glands adrenals parathyroids	White	Black	G	D
Element wood	White (GB)	Green (Li)	G (GB)	A (Li)

114

Spasm

Sudden, violent involuntary contraction of one or more muscles.
Ear points: Affected area and 35, 19 int., 21.

STEPS	COLORS		SOUNDS	
	V-Out **A-In**	**In** **Out**	**A-Out** **V-In**	**In** **Out**
Area affected area	Green	Yellow	A	F
Glands parathyroids	White	Black	G	D
Element water	Blue (Bl)	Yellow (Ki)	D (Bl)	F (Ki)

Torticollis (wryneck)

Painful twisting or contraction of the neck muscles resulting in altered
carriage of the head.
Ear points: Massage the area of the cervical spine shown in figure 17,
page 97.

STEPS	COLORS		SOUNDS	
	V-Out **A-In**	**In** **Out**	**A-Out** **V-In**	**In** **Out**
Area neck	Green	Yellow	A	F
Glands adrenals	White	Black	G	D
Elements water wood	Blue (Bl) White (GB)	Yellow (Ki) Green (Li)	D (Bl) G (GB)	F (Ki) A (Li)

The Nervous System and the Psyche

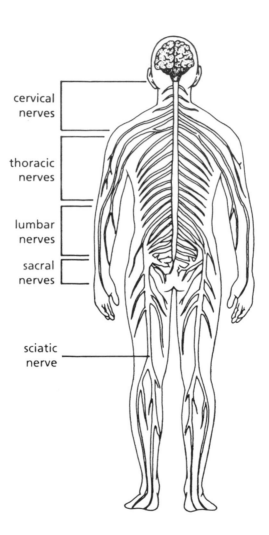

cervical
nerves

thoracic
nerves

lumbar
nerves

sacral
nerves

sciatic
nerve

Alcoholism

Abuse of alcoholic beverages leading to a variety of problems.
Ear points: 16, 35, 21, 11.

STEPS	COLORS		SOUNDS	
	V-Out **A-In**	**In** **Out**	**A-Out** **V-In**	**In** **Out**
Area hypothalamus	Green	Yellow	A	F
Glands pancreas adrenals pituitary	White	Black	G	D
Elements				
wood	White (GB)	Green (Li)	G (GB)	A (Li)
fire	Blue (SI)	Red (Ht)	D (SI)	C (Ht)

Anorexia

Seek medical attention

Reduction or loss of appetite.
Ear points: 33, 6, 11.

STEPS	COLORS		SOUNDS	
	V-Out **A-In**	**In** **Out**	**A-Out** **V-In**	**In** **Out**
Area hypothalamus	Green	Yellow	A	F
Glands gonads pancreas thyroid	White	Black	G	D
Elements				
wood	White (GB)	Green (Li)	G (GB)	A (Li)
fire	Blue (SI)	Red (Ht)	D (SI)	C (Ht)

Anxiety

Mental or physical disorder characterized by strong fear or apprehension
and feelings of constriction.
Ear points: 35, 19 ext., 21.

STEPS	COLORS		SOUNDS	
	V-Out **A-In**	**In** **Out**	**A-Out** **V-In**	**In** **Out**
Area hypothalamus	Green	Yellow	A	F
Glands pancreas adrenals thymus	White	Black	G	D
Elements wood metal	White (GB) White (Co)	Green (Li) Red (Lu)	G (GB) G (Co)	A (Li) C (Lu)

Ataxia

Inability to coordinate voluntary muscles due to a dysfunction of the
nervous system.
Ear points: 28, 19 ext., 22, 14.

STEPS	COLORS		SOUNDS	
	V-Out **A-In**	**In** **Out**	**A-Out** **V-In**	**In** **Out**
Area solar plexus brain	Green	Yellow	A	F
Glands entire endo- crine system	White	Black	G	D
Elements water	Blue (Bl)	Yellow (Ki)	D (Bl)	F (Ki)

Bulimia

Seek medical attention

Exaggerated feeling of hunger with an irrisistible need to eat large quantities of food and then vomit to purge the system.
Ear points: 16, 17, 1, 6, 26 int. and ext., 21.

STEPS	COLORS		SOUNDS	
	V-Out **A-In**	**In** **Out**	**A-Out** **V-In**	**In** **Out**
Area hypothalamus	Green	Yellow	A	F
Glands gonads pancreas thyroid	White	Black	G	D
Elements wood fire	White (GB) Blue (SI)	Green (Li) Red (Ht)	G (GB) D (SI)	A (Li) C (Ht)

Depression

Drop in energy level accompanied by sadness and negative thoughts.
Ear points: 1, 2, 5, 19 ext., 21, 25.

STEPS	COLORS		SOUNDS	
	V-Out **A-In**	**In** **Out**	**A-Out** **V-In**	**In** **Out**
Area brain	Green	Yellow	A	F
Glands adrenals thyroid pituitary pineal	White	Black	G	D
Elements metal water wood	White (Co) Blue (Bl) White (GB)	Red (Lu) Yellow (Ki) Green (Li)	G (Co) D (Bl) G (GB)	C (Lu) F (Ki) A (Li)

119

Emotional instability

Alternation of moods between depression and agitation.
Ear points: 17, 26 ext., 21.

STEPS	COLORS		SOUNDS	
	V-Out **A-In**	**In** **Out**	**A-Out** **V-In**	**In** **Out**
Area solar plexus brain	Green	Yellow	A	F
Glands adrenals thyroid	White	Black	G	D
Elements metal water	White (Co) Blue (Bl)	Red (Lu) Yellow (Ki)	G (Co) D (Bl)	C (Lu) F (Ki)

Encephalitis

Seek medical attention

Inflammation of the brain.
Ear points: 35, 34, 27, 28.

STEPS	COLORS		SOUNDS	
	V-Out **A-In**	**In** **Out**	**A-Out** **V-In**	**In** **Out**
Area brain	Green	Yellow	A	F
Glands entire endo- crine system	White	Black	G	D
Element wood	White (GB)	Green (Li)	G (GB)	A (Li)

Epilepsy

Seek medical attention

Nervous system disorder characterized by convulsions with loss of consciousness.

Ear points: 17, 26 int., 22.

STEPS	COLORS		SOUNDS	
	V-Out **A-In**	**In** **Out**	**A-Out** **V-In**	**In** **Out**
Area brain	Green	Yellow	A	F
Glands entire endocrine system	White	Black	G	D
Elements				
metal	White (Co)	Red (Lu)	G (Co)	C (Lu)
water	Blue (Bl)	Yellow (Ki)	D (Bl)	F (Ki)

Headache, migraine

Head pain, usually caused by a disturbance of the meridians of the gallbladder or bladder, or tension in the neck muscles.

Ear points: 1, 17, 27, 9, 11.

STEPS	COLORS		SOUNDS	
	V-Out **A-In**	**In** **Out**	**A-Out** **V-In**	**In** **Out**
Area brain	Green	Yellow	A	F
Gland pituitary	White	Black	G	D
Elements				
water	Blue (Bl)	Yellow (Ki)	D (Bl)	F (Ki)
wood	White (GB)	Green (Li)	G (GB)	A (Li)

Hiccups

Spasms of the diaphragm.
Ear points: 1, 6, 21.

STEPS	COLORS		SOUNDS	
	V-Out A-In	In Out	A-Out V-In	In Out
Area diaphragm	Green	Yellow	A	F
Glands adrenals	White	Black	G	D
Element metal	White (Co)	Red (Lu)	G (Co)	C (Lu)

Insomnia

Difficulty in getting sufficient sleep.
Ear points: 1, 3, 21, 24.

STEPS	COLORS		SOUNDS	
	V-Out A-In	In Out	A-Out V-In	In Out
Area hypothalamus	Green	Yellow	A	F
Glands adrenals pituitary pineal	White	Black	G	D
Elements metal	White (Co)	Red (Lu)	G (Co)	C (Lu)
wood	White (GB)	Green (Li)	G (GB)	A (Li)

Meningitis

Seek medical attention

Inflammation of the meninges (membranes surrounding the brain and spinal cord).
Ear points: 26 int., 35, 28.

STEPS	COLORS		SOUNDS	
	V-Out A-In	In Out	A-Out V-In	In Out
Area brain	Green	Yellow	A	F
Glands adrenals thymus pituitary pineal	White	Black	G	D
Elements				
water	Blue (Bl)	Yellow (Ki)	D (Bl)	F (Ki)
wood	White (GB)	Green (Li)	G (GB)	A (Li)

Multiple sclerosis

Seek medical attention

Deterioration of the nerves' myelin coat.
Ear points: 28, 19 ext., 22, 14.

STEPS	COLORS		SOUNDS	
	V-Out A-In	In Out	A-Out V-In	In Out
Area entire ner- vous system	Green	Yellow	A	F
Glands entire endo- crine system	White	Black	G	D
Elements				
metal	White (Co)	Red (Lu)	G (Co)	C (Lu)
water	Blue (Bl)	Yellow (Ki)	D (Bl)	F (Ki)

Nervous tension

Irritability and poor response to stress.
Ear points: 17, 26 int. and ext., 21.

STEPS	COLORS		SOUNDS	
	V-Out **A-In**	**In** **Out**	**A-Out** **V-In**	**In** **Out**
Area solar plexus brain	Green	Yellow	A	F
Glands adrenals	White	Black	G	D
Elements				
metal	White (Co)	Red (Lu)	G (Co)	C (Lu)
water	Blue (Bl)	Yellow (Ki)	D (Bl)	F (Ki)
wood	White (GB)	Green (Li)	G (GB)	A (Li)

Neuralgia

Pain felt along a sensory nerve.
Ear points: Affected area and 16, 28, 23.

STEPS	COLORS		SOUNDS	
	V-Out **A-In**	**In** **Out**	**A-Out** **V-In**	**In** **Out**
Area affected area	Green	Yellow	A	F
Glands adrenals pituitary	White	Black	G	D
Elements				
water	Blue (Bl)	Yellow (Ki)	D (Bl)	F (Ki)
metal	White (Co)	Red (Lu)	G (Co)	C (Lu)
wood	White (GB)	Green (Li)	G (GB)	A (Li)

Neuritis

Inflammation of a nerve, sometimes accompanied by degenerative changes in the nerve.

Ear points: Affected area and 16, 28, 23.

STEPS	COLORS		SOUNDS	
	V-Out **A-In**	**In** **Out**	**A-Out** **V-In**	**In** **Out**
Area affected nerve	Green	Yellow	A	F
Glands adrenals thymus	White	Black	G	D
Element water	Blue (Bl)	Yellow (Ki)	D (Bl)	F (Ki)

Nightmares

Distressing dreams.

Ear points: 1, 17, 27.

STEPS	COLORS		SOUNDS	
	V-Out **A-In**	**In** **Out**	**A-Out** **V-In**	**In** **Out**
Area hypothalamus	Green	Yellow	A	F
Glands pancreas pineal	White	Black	G	D
Element wood	White (GB)	Green (Li)	G (GB)	A (Li)

125

Paralysis

Seek medical attention

Loss of motor function due to lesions of the nervous system.
Ear points: 26 int. and ext., 30, 19 ext.

Steps	Colors		Sounds	
	V-Out **A-In**	**In** **Out**	**A-Out** **V-In**	**In** **Out**
Area affected area	Green	Yellow	A	F
Gland pituitary	White	Black	G	D
Elements water wood	 Blue (Bl) White (GB)	 Yellow (Ki) Green (Li)	 D (Bl) G (GB)	 F (Ki) A (Li)

Paresis of the Hand

Feeling of stiffness and numbness in the fingers.
Ear points: 26 int., 30, 28. Also massage the area of the hand shown in
  figure 17, page 97.

Steps	Colors		Sounds	
	V-Out **A-In**	**In** **Out**	**A-Out** **V-In**	**In** **Out**
Area fingers	Green	Yellow	A	F
Glands adrenals pituitary	White	Black	G	D
Elements metal water	 White (Co) Blue (Bl)	 Red (Lu) Yellow (Ki)	 G (Co) D (Bl)	 C (Lu) F (Ki)

Parkinson's disease

Progressive disease of the nervous system, which causes muscular trembling.

Ear points: 26 int. and ext., 30, 28, 14.

STEPS	COLORS		SOUNDS	
	V-Out **A-In**	**In** **Out**	**A-Out** **V-In**	**In** **Out**
Area nervous system	Green	Yellow	A	F
Glands entire endo- crine system	White	Black	G	D
Elements				
metal	White (Co)	Red (Lu)	G (Co)	C (Lu)
water	Blue (Bl)	Yellow (Ki)	D (Bl)	F (Ki)

Sciatica

Inflammation of the body's longest nerve, which starts at the sacral plexus and runs through the pelvis to the heel.

Ear points: 26 ext., 22, 13, 25.

STEPS	COLORS		SOUNDS	
	V-Out **A-In**	**In** **Out**	**A-Out** **V-In**	**In** **Out**
Area sciatic nerve	Green	Yellow	A	F
Glands adrenals thymus	White	Black	G	D
Element				
water	Blue (Bl)	Yellow (Ki)	D (Bl)	F (Ki)

Stuttering

Difficulty in speaking fluently.
Ear points: 26 int. and ext., 27, 21.

STEPS	COLORS		SOUNDS	
	V-Out **A-In**	**In** **Out**	**A-Out** **V-In**	**In** **Out**
Area brain	Green	Yellow	A	F
Gland thyroid	White	Black	G	D
Elements				
water	Blue (Bl)	Yellow (Ki)	D (Bl)	F (Ki)
wood	White (GB)	Green (Li)	G (GB)	A (Li)

Trembling

Involuntary movements of the body.
Ear points: 26 int. and ext., 30, 28, 14.

STEPS	COLORS		SOUNDS	
	V-Out **A-In**	**In** **Out**	**A-Out** **V-In**	**In** **Out**
Area entire nervous system	Green	Yellow	A	F
Glands adrenals thyroid	White	Black	G	D
Elements				
metal	White (Co)	Red (Lu)	G (Co)	C (Lu)
water	Blue (Bl)	Yellow (Ki)	D (Bl)	F (Ki)

Twitching

Short, involuntary, and repeated spastic contraction or jerking movement.

Ear points: 26 int. and ext., 30, 21.

STEPS	COLORS		SOUNDS	
	V-Out **A-In**	**In** **Out**	**A-Out** **V-In**	**In** **Out**
Area solar plexus brain	Green	Yellow	A	F
Glands adrenals	White	Black	G	D
Elements				
metal	White (GB)	Red (Lu)	G (GB)	C (Lu)
water	Blue (Bl)	Yellow (Ki)	D (Bl)	F (Ki)

Vertigo

Dizziness, which can be accompanied by loss of equilibrium.

Ear points: 3, 34, and zones between 28 and 29. Also massage the area of the cervical spine shown in figure 17, page 97.

STEPS	COLORS		SOUNDS	
	V-Out **A-In**	**In** **Out**	**A-Out** **V-In**	**In** **Out**
Area middle and inner ear brain	Green	Yellow	A	F
Glands gonads pancreas thyroid	White	Black	G	D
Elements				
water	Blue (Bl)	Yellow (Ki)	D (Bl)	F (Ki)
wood	White (GB)	Green (Li)	G (GB)	A (Li)

The Endocrine System

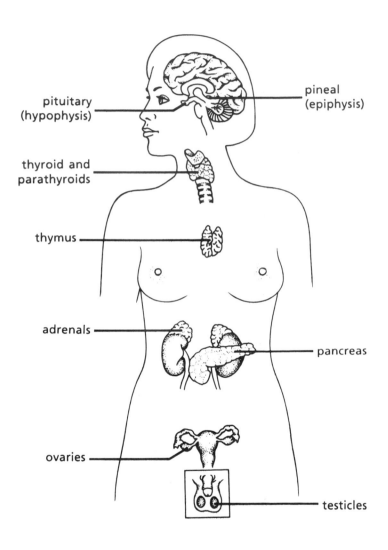

pituitary
(hypophysis)

pineal
(epiphysis)

thyroid and
parathyroids

thymus

adrenals

pancreas

ovaries

testicles

Allergies

Abnormal inflammatory reaction to specific substances (foods, fabrics or other environmental matter) to which the individual is sensitive.
Ear points: 19 int., 21, 24.

STEPS	COLORS		SOUNDS	
	V-Out **A-In**	**In** **Out**	**A-Out** **V-In**	**In** **Out**
Area affected area	Green	Yellow	A	F
Glands pancreas adrenals	White	Black	G	D
Elements wood metal	White (GB) White (Co)	Green (Li) Red (Lu)	G (GB) G (Co)	A (Li) C (Lu)

Chills

Difficulty in retaining body heat.
Ear points: 34, 27, 11, 15.

STEPS	COLORS		SOUNDS	
	V-Out **A-In**	**In** **Out**	**A-Out** **V-In**	**In** **Out**
Area hypothalamus	Green	Yellow	A	F
Glands gonads adrenals thyroid	White	Black	G	D
Element wood	White (GB)	Green (Li)	G (GB)	A (Li)

Diabetes

Seek medical attention

Chronic metabolic dysfunction generated by inadequate insulin secretion.

Ear points: 33, 9, 11.

STEPS	COLORS		SOUNDS	
	V-Out **A-In**	**In** **Out**	**A-Out** **V-In**	**In** **Out**
Area pancreas	Green	Yellow	A	F
Glands pancreas adrenals pituitary	White	Black	G	D
Element wood	White (GB)	Green (Li)	G (GB)	A (Li)

Excessive thinness

Inadequate weight.

Ear points: 26 int. and ext., 27, 11.

STEPS	COLORS		SOUNDS	
	V-Out **A-In**	**In** **Out**	**A-Out** **V-In**	**In** **Out**
Area hypothalamus	Green	Yellow	A	F
Gland thyroid	White	Black	G	D
Elements wood fire	White (GB) Blue (SI)	Green (Li) Red (Ht)	G (GB) D (SI)	A (Li) C (Ht)

Goiter

Enlargement of the thyroid gland.
Ear points: 26, 6, 21.

STEPS	COLORS		SOUNDS	
	V-Out **A-In**	**In** **Out**	**A-Out** **V-In**	**In** **Out**
Area hypothalamus	Green	Yellow	A	F
Gland thyroid	White	Black	G	D
Element fire	Blue (SI)	Red (Ht)	D (SI)	C (Ht)

Hypoglycemia

Seek medical attention

Inadequate blood sugar level caused by excessive insulin secretion.
Ear points: 33, 6, 21, 9.

STEPS	COLORS		SOUNDS	
	V-Out **A-In**	**In** **Out**	**A-Out** **V-In**	**In** **Out**
Area hypothalamus	Green	Yellow	A	F
Glands pancreas adrenals pituitary	White	Black	G	D
Element wood	White (GB)	Green (Li)	G (GB)	A (Li)

Obesity

Excessive weight.
Ear points: 27, 21, 32.

STEPS	COLORS		SOUNDS	
	V-Out **A-In**	**In** **Out**	**A-Out** **V-In**	**In** **Out**
Area hypothalamus	Green	Yellow	A	F
Glands gonads thyroid pituitary	White	Black	G	D
Element wood	White (GB)	Green (Li)	G (GB)	A (Li)

Premature aging

Unusually early appearance of the characteristics of old age.
Ear points: 26 int. and ext., 6, 21.

STEPS	COLORS		SOUNDS	
	V-Out **A-In**	**In** **Out**	**A-Out** **V-In**	**In** **Out**
Area hypothalamus	Green	Yellow	A	F
Glands entire endo- crine system	White	Black	G	D
Element wood	White (GB)	Green (Li)	G (GB)	A (Li)

134

Stress

Body's response to negative physiological and psychological factors.
Ear points: 26 ext., 19 ext., 21, 13.

STEPS	COLORS		SOUNDS	
	V-Out **A-In**	**In** **Out**	**A-Out** **V-In**	**In** **Out**
Area solar plexus brain	Green	Yellow	A	F
Glands adrenals	White	Black	G	D
Elements metal water	White (Co) Blue (Bl)	Red (Lu) Yellow (Ki)	G (Co) D (Bl)	C (Lu) F (Ki)

The Lymphatic System

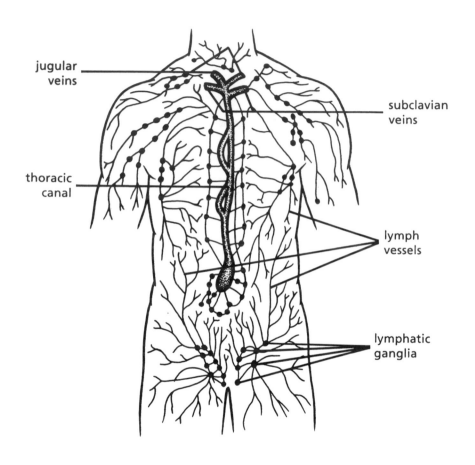

jugular
veins

subclavian
veins

thoracic
canal

lymph
vessels

lymphatic
ganglia

Abscess

Accumulation of pus, which forms a pocket in a tissue or an organ.
Ear points: Affected area and 35, 11.

STEPS	COLORS		SOUNDS	
	V-Out **A-In**	**In** **Out**	**A-Out** **V-In**	**In** **Out**
Area affected area	Green	Yellow	A	F
Glands pancreas adrenals thymus	White	Black	G	D
Element wood	White (GB)	Green (Li)	G (GB)	A (Li)

Adenoidal swelling

Enlargement of the pharyngeal tonsil, located behind the nasal cavity.
Ear points: 2, 35, 7.

STEPS	COLORS		SOUNDS	
	V-Out **A-In**	**In** **Out**	**A-Out** **V-In**	**In** **Out**
Area behind nasal cavity	Green	Yellow	A	F
Glands adrenals thymus pituitary	White	Black	G	D
Element wood	White (GB)	Green (Li)	G (GB)	A (Li)

Cellulitis

Inflammation of the subcutaneous cellular tissue.
Ear points: 26 int., 19 int., 21, 15, 24.

STEPS	COLORS		SOUNDS	
	V-Out **A-In**	**In** **Out**	**A-Out** **V-In**	**In** **Out**
Area affected area	Green	Yellow	A	F
Glands gonads thymus thyroid	White	Black	G	D
Elements water wood	Blue (Bl) White (GB)	Yellow (Ki) Green (Li)	D (Bl) G (GB)	F (Ki) A (Li)

Edema

Seek medical attention

Diffuse swelling caused by an inordinate accumulation of liquid in connective tissue.
Ear points: Affected area and 15, 24.

STEPS	COLORS		SOUNDS	
	V-Out **A-In**	**In** **Out**	**A-Out** **V-In**	**In** **Out**
Area affected area	Green	Yellow	A	F
Glands gonads adrenals pituitary	White	Black	G	D
Elements water wood	Blue (Bl) White (GB)	Yellow (Ki) Green (Li)	D (Bl) G (GB)	F (Ki) A (Li)

Flu

Infectious viral illness whose symptoms include fever, stiffness, and respiratory tract problems.

Ear points: 2, 35, 24.

STEPS	COLORS		SOUNDS	
	V-Out **A-In**	**In** **Out**	**A-Out** **V-In**	**In** **Out**
Area hypothalamus	Green	Yellow	A	F
Glands thymus thyroid pituitary	White	Black	G	D
Element wood	White (GB)	Green (Li)	G (GB)	A (Li)

Infection

Illness or inflammation resulting from bacteria or viruses entering the body.

Ear points: Affected area and 35.

STEPS	COLORS		SOUNDS	
	V-Out **A-In**	**In** **Out**	**A-Out** **V-In**	**In** **Out**
Area affected area	Green	Yellow	A	F
Glands adrenals thymus	White	Black	G	D
Element wood	White (GB)	Green (Li)	G (GB)	A (Li)

Inflammation

Redness, swelling, and pain of the affected part—the body's natural
reaction as it attempts to heal itself.
Ear points: Affected area and 35.

Steps	Colors		Sounds	
	V-Out **A-In**	**In** **Out**	**A-Out** **V-In**	**In** **Out**
Area affected area	Green	Yellow	A	F
Glands adrenals pituitary	White	Black	G	D
Element wood	White (GB)	Green (Li)	G (GB)	A (Li)

Leukemia

Seek medical attention

Disease characterized by increased leukocytes in the blood and the proliferation of lymphatic tissue cells.
Ear points: 21, 15, 24.

Steps	Colors		Sounds	
	V-Out **A-In**	**In** **Out**	**A-Out** **V-In**	**In** **Out**
Area spleen	Green	Yellow	A	F
Glands entire endo- crine system	White	Black	G	D
Element wood	White (GB)	Green (Li)	G (GB)	A (Li)

140

Tonsillitis

Inflammation of the palatine tonsils.
Ear points: 1, 35, 34, 7.

STEPS	COLORS		SOUNDS	
	V-Out **A-In**	**In** **Out**	**A-Out** **V-In**	**In** **Out**
Area tonsils	Green	Yellow	A	F
Glands adrenals thymus	White	Black	G	D
Element wood	White (GB)	Green (Li)	G (GB)	A (Li)

The Cardiovascular System

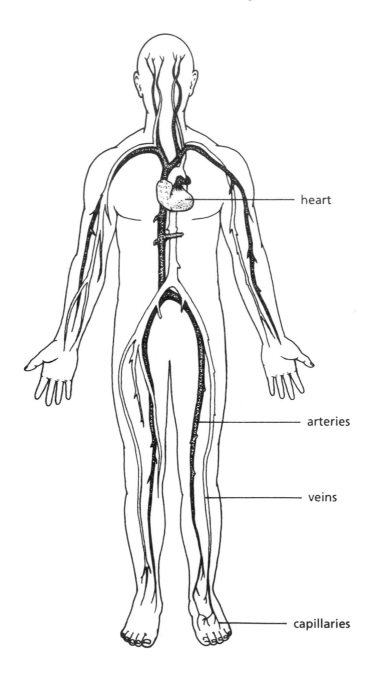

heart

arteries

veins

capillaries

Anemia

Low red blood cell count and hemoglobin content.
Ear points: 6, 9, 11.

STEPS	COLORS		SOUNDS	
	V-Out **A-In**	**In** **Out**	**A-Out** **V-In**	**In** **Out**
Area spleen	Green	Yellow	A	F
Gland thyroid	White	Black	G	D
Element wood	White (GB)	Green (Li)	G (GB)	A (Li)

Aneurysm

Seek medical attention

Abnormal dilation of the wall of a blood vessel or heart cavity.
Ear points: 26 int. and ext., 21.

STEPS	COLORS		SOUNDS	
	V-Out **A-In**	**In** **Out**	**A-Out** **V-In**	**In** **Out**
Area affected area	Green	Yellow	A	F
Glands entire endo- crine system	White	Black	G	D
Element fire	Blue (SI)	Red (Ht)	D (SI)	C (Ht)

Angina pectoris

Seek medical attention

Spasm affecting the muscles of the heart.
Ear points: 26 int. and ext., 28, 21, 24.

STEPS	COLORS		SOUNDS	
	V-Out **A-In**	**In** **Out**	**A-Out** **V-In**	**In** **Out**
Area heart solar plexus	Green	Yellow	A	F
Glands pancreas adrenals thyroid	White	Black	G	D
Elements				
metal	White (Co)	Red (Lu)	G (Co)	C (Lu)
water	Blue (Bl)	Yellow (Ki)	D (Bl)	F (Ki)

Arteriosclerosis; Atheroma

Seek medical attention

Hardening of the arteries; fatty deposits in the arteries.
Ear points: 26 int. and ext., 21, 25, 24.

STEPS	COLORS		SOUNDS	
	V-Out **A-In**	**In** **Out**	**A-Out** **V-In**	**In** **Out**
Area affected area	Green	Yellow	A	F
Glands gonads adrenals thyroid	White	Black	G	D
Element wood	White (GB)	Green (Li)	G (GB)	A (Li)

Arrhythmia

Seek medical attention

Irregular heartbeat.
Ear points: 16, 26 int. and ext., 28, 21.

STEPS	COLORS		SOUNDS	
	V-Out **A-In**	**In** **Out**	**A-Out** **V-In**	**In** **Out**
Area hypothalamus	Green	Yellow	A	F
Glands adrenals pituitary	White	Black	G	D
Elements				
fire	Blue (SI)	Red (Ht)	D (SI)	C (Ht)
metal	White (Co)	Red (Lu)	G (Co)	C (Lu)
water	Blue (Bl)	Yellow (Ki)	D (Bl)	F (Ki)

Bradycardia

Seek medical attention

Relatively slow heart action (less than 60 beats per minute).
Ear points: 35, 34, 6.

STEPS	COLORS		SOUNDS	
	V-Out **A-In**	**In** **Out**	**A-Out** **V-In**	**In** **Out**
Area hypothalamus	Green	Yellow	A	F
Glands adrenals thyroid pituitary	White	Black	G	D
Elements				
fire	Blue (SI)	Red (Ht)	D (SI)	C (Ht)
water	Blue (Bl)	Yellow (Ki)	D (Bl)	F (Ki)

Cerebral hemorrhage

Seek medical attention

Heavy discharge of blood from the arteries of the brain, provoking paralysis, loss of consciousness, and possible brain damage.
Ear points: 1, 26 int., 21.

Steps	Colors		Sounds	
	V-Out **A-In**	**In** **Out**	**A-Out** **V-In**	**In** **Out**
Area brain	Green	Yellow	A	F
Glands parathyroids pituitary	White	Black	G	D
Element wood	White (GB)	Green (Li)	G (GB)	A (Li)

Coronary occlusion

Seek medical attention

Obstruction of an artery to the heart caused by arteriosclerosis, an embolism, or thrombosis.
Ear points: 26 int., 28, 19 int.

Steps	Colors		Sounds	
	V-Out **A-In**	**In** **Out**	**A-Out** **V-In**	**In** **Out**
Area heart solar plexus	Green	Yellow	A	F
Glands entire endo- crine system	White	Black	G	D
Elements metal water	White (Co) Blue (Bl)	Red (Lu) Yellow (Ki)	G (Co) D (Bl)	C (Lu) F (Ki)

High cholesterol

Seek medical attention

Abnormally high level of cholesterol in the body (brain, blood plasma, bile) which can lead to arteriosclerosis and gallstones.
Ear points: 26 ext., 11, 32.

STEPS	COLORS		SOUNDS	
	V-Out **A-In**	**In** **Out**	**A-Out** **V-In**	**In** **Out**
Area entire circu- latory system	Green	Yellow	A	F
Gland thyroid	White	Black	G	D
Element wood	White (GB)	Green (Li)	G (GB)	A (Li)

Hypertension

Seek medical attention

Above-normal blood pressure.
Ear points: 17, 21, 8 , 24.

STEPS	COLORS		SOUNDS	
	V-Out **A-In**	**In** **Out**	**A-Out** **V-In**	**In** **Out**
Area hypothalamus	Green	Yellow	A	F
Glands adrenals thyroid pituitary	White	Black	G	D
Elements water metal	Blue (Bl) White (Co)	Yellow (Ki) Red (Lu)	D (Bl) G (Co)	F (Ki) C (Lu)

Hypotension

Seek medical attention

Below-normal blood pressure.
Ear points: 26 ext., 34, 35, 27.

STEPS	COLORS		SOUNDS	
	V-Out **A-In**	**In** **Out**	**A-Out** **V-In**	**In** **Out**
Area hypothalamus	Green	Yellow	A	F
Glands adrenals thyroid pituitary	White	Black	G	D
Elements				
water	Blue (Bl)	Yellow (Ki)	D (Bl)	F (Ki)
metal	White (Co)	Red (Lu)	G (Co)	C (Lu)

Myocardial infarction

Seek medical attention

Necrosis of part of the heart muscle.
Ear points: 16, 26 int., 21, 24, 10.

STEPS	COLORS		SOUNDS	
	V-Out **A-In**	**In** **Out**	**A-Out** **V-In**	**In** **Out**
Area heart solar plexus	Green	Yellow	A	F
Glands adrenals	White	Black	G	D
Elements				
fire	Blue (SI)	Red (Ht)	D (SI)	C (Ht)
metal	White (Co)	Red (Lu)	G (Co)	C (Lu)

Phlebitis

Seek medical attention

Inflammation of a vein accompanied by the formation of a blood clot, often in the leg.

Ear points: 35, 11, 25.

STEPS	COLORS			SOUNDS	
	V-Out **A-In**	**In** **Out**		**A-Out** **V-In**	**In** **Out**
Area affected area	Green	Yellow		A	F
Glands gonads adrenals thyroid	White	Black		G	D
Elements wood metal	White (GB) White (Co)	Green (Li) Red (Lu)		G (GB) G (Co)	A (Li) C (Lu)

Raynaud's disease

Spasms affecting the dilation of blood vessels in the body's extremities.
Ear points: 16, 1, 28, 21.

STEPS	COLORS			SOUNDS	
	V-Out **A-In**	**In** **Out**		**A-Out** **V-In**	**In** **Out**
Area hypothalamus	Green	Yellow		A	F
Glands gonads adrenals thyroid	White	Black		G	D
Elements fire wood	Blue (SI) White (GB)	Red (Ht) Green (Li)		D (SI) G (GB)	C (Ht) A (Li)

149

Rheumatic fever

Seek medical attention

Inflammation of the membrane around the heart and also of the connective tissue around the joints.
Ear points: 1, 26 int., 25, 21, 11.

STEPS	COLORS		SOUNDS	
	V-Out **A-In**	**In** **Out**	**A-Out** **V-In**	**In** **Out**
Area heart connective tissue around the inflamed joints	Green	Yellow	A	F
Glands gonads adrenals thymus thyroid pituitary	White	Black	G	D
Element fire	Blue (SI)	Red (Ht)	D (SI)	C (Ht)

Tachycardia

Accelerated heartbeat.
Ear points: 26 ext., 34, 21, 24.

STEPS	COLORS		SOUNDS	
	V-Out **A-In**	**In** **Out**	**A-Out** **V-In**	**In** **Out**
Area hypothalamus	Green	Yellow	A	F
Glands adrenals thyroid	White	Black	G	D
Elements metal water	White (Co) Blue (Bl)	Red (Lu) Yellow (Ki)	G (Co) D (Bl)	C (Lu) F (Ki)

Thrombosis

Seek medical attention

Formation of a clot in a blood vessel or one of the heart's cavities.
Ear points: 35, 11, 25.

STEPS	COLORS		SOUNDS	
	V-Out **A-In**	**In** **Out**	**A-Out** **V-In**	**In** **Out**
Area affected area	Green	Yellow	A	F
Glands adrenals parathyroids	White	Black	G	D
Element wood	White (GB)	Green (Li)	G (GB)	A (Li)

Varicose veins

Permanent dilation of a vein.
Ear points: 22, 14, 25.

STEPS	COLORS		SOUNDS	
	V-Out **A-In**	**In** **Out**	**A-Out** **V-In**	**In** **Out**
Area affected area	Green	Yellow	A	F
Glands pancreas adrenals thyroid pituitary	White	Black	G	D
Elements wood	White (GB)	Green (Li)	G (GB)	A (Li)
metal	White (Co)	Red (Lu)	G (Co)	C (Lu)
fire	Blue (SI)	Red (Ht)	D (SI)	C (Ht)

The Respiratory System

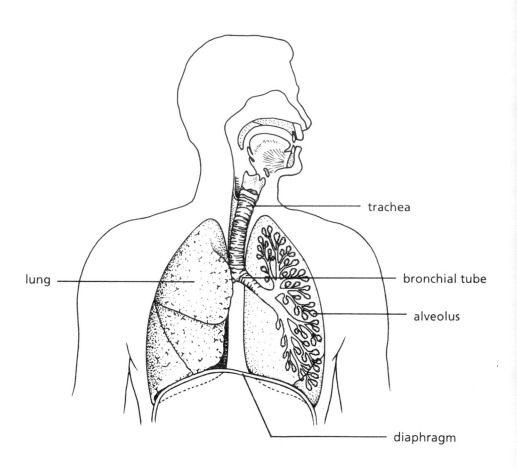

trachea

lung

bronchial tube

alveolus

diaphragm

Asthma

Seek medical attention

Bronchial spasm interfering with breathing and often accompanied by increased bronchial secretions.
Ear points: 34, 4, 24.

STEPS	COLORS		SOUNDS	
	V-Out **A-In**	**In** **Out**	**A-Out** **V-In**	**In** **Out**
Area entire respira- tory system hypothalamus	Green	Yellow	A	F
Glands adrenals	White	Black	G	D
Elements metal wood	White (Co) White (GB)	Red (Lu) Green (Li)	G (Co) G (GB)	C (Lu) A (Li)

Bronchitis

Inflammation of the mucous membrane of the bronchi.
Ear points: 35, 34, 4, 24.

STEPS	COLORS		SOUNDS	
	V-Out **A-In**	**In** **Out**	**A-Out** **V-In**	**In** **Out**
Area respiratory passageway	Green	Yellow	A	F
Glands adrenals thymus	White	Black	G	D
Elements metal wood	White (Co) White (GB)	Red (Lu) Green (Li)	G (Co) G (GB)	C (Lu) A (Li)

Cold

Acute inflammation of the nasal mucous membrane.
Ear points: 2, 5, 7, 24.

STEPS	COLORS		SOUNDS	
	V-Out **A-In**	**In** **Out**	**A-Out** **V-In**	**In** **Out**
Area throat nose sinus eyes	Green	Yellow	A	F
Glands adrenals thymus	White	Black	G	D
Elements metal	White (Co)	Red (Lu)	G (Co)	C (Lu)
wood	White (GB)	Green (Li)	G (GB)	A (Li)

Croup

Seek medical attention

Spasm of the larynx, especially in children, characterized by difficulty in
  breathing and a loud cough.
Ear points: 4, 19 int., 21.

STEPS	COLORS		SOUNDS	
	V-Out **A-In**	**In** **Out**	**A-Out** **V-In**	**In** **Out**
Area hypothalamus	Green	Yellow	A	F
Glands adrenals	White	Black	G	D
Elements metal	White (Co)	Red (Lu)	G (Co)	C (Lu)
water	Blue (Bl)	Yellow (Ki)	D (Bl)	F (Ki)

154

Hay fever

Allergic reaction affecting the conjunctiva of the eyes, the nasal mucous
   membranes, and the sinuses.
Ear points: 34, 21, 24.

STEPS	COLORS		SOUNDS	
	V-Out **A-In**	**In** **Out**	**A-Out** **V-In**	**In** **Out**
Area eyes nose sinus	Green	Yellow	A	F
Glands adrenals	White	Black	G	D
Elements metal wood	White (Co) White (GB)	Red (Lu) Green (Li)	G (Co) G (GB)	C (Lu) A (Li)

Laryngitis, pharyngitis

Inflammation of the larynx or pharynx.
Ear points: 1, 35, 34, 7.

STEPS	COLORS		SOUNDS	
	V-Out **A-In**	**In** **Out**	**A-Out** **V-In**	**In** **Out**
Area larynx pharynx	Green	Yellow	A	F
Glands adrenals thymus	White	Black	G	D
Element wood	White (GB)	Green (Li)	G (GB)	A (Li)

Nicotine-related ailments

Various physiological and mental disorders caused by nicotine abuse.
Ear points: 2, 17, 21.

STEPS	COLORS		SOUNDS	
	V-Out **A-In**	**In** **Out**	**A-Out** **V-In**	**In** **Out**
Area hypothalamus	Green	Yellow	A	F
Glands gonads adrenals thyroid	White	Black	G	D
Elements				
metal	White (Co)	Red (Lu)	G (Co)	C (Lu)
water	Blue (Bl)	Yellow (Ki)	D (Bl)	F (Ki)

Pleurisy

Seek medical attention

Inflammation of the pleura, the membrane covering the lungs.
Ear points: 26 int., 4, 19 int.

STEPS	COLORS		SOUNDS	
	V-Out **A-In**	**In** **Out**	**A-Out** **V-In**	**In** **Out**
Area lungs	Green	Yellow	A	F
Glands adrenals	White	Black	G	D
Element wood	White (GB)	Green (Li)	G (GB)	A (Li)

Pneumonia

Seek medical attention

Acute inflammation of the lungs.
Ear points: 26 int., 4, 5, 19 int.

STEPS	COLORS		SOUNDS	
	V-Out **A-In**	**In** **Out**	**A-Out** **V-In**	**In** **Out**
Area lungs	Green	Yellow	A	F
Glands entire endo- crine system	White	Black	G	D
Elements metal	White (Co)	Red (Lu)	G (Co)	C (Lu)
wood	White (GB)	Green (Li)	G (GB)	A (Li)

Pulmonary emphysema

Seek medical attention

Permanent dilation of the pulmonary alveoli, causing a chronic cough.
Ear points: 26 int., 4, 5, 19 int.

STEPS	COLORS		SOUNDS	
	V-Out **A-In**	**In** **Out**	**A-Out** **V-In**	**In** **Out**
Area lungs	Green	Yellow	A	F
Glands adrenals	White	Black	G	D
Element wood	White (GB)	Green (Li)	G (GB)	A (Li)

Rhinitis

Inflammation of the mucous membrane of the nose.
Ear points: 2, 35, 21.

STEPS	COLORS		SOUNDS	
	V-Out **A-In**	**In** **Out**	**A-Out** **V-In**	**In** **Out**
Area nasal cavities	Green	Yellow	A	F
Glands thymus pituitary	White	Black	G	D
Elements metal wood	White (Co) White (GB)	Red (Lu) Green (Li)	G (Co) G (GB)	C (Lu) A (Li)

Sinusitis

Inflammation of the sinuses.
Ear points: 2, 35, 21.

STEPS	COLORS		SOUNDS	
	V-Out **A-In**	**In** **Out**	**A-Out** **V-In**	**In** **Out**
Area sinuses	Green	Yellow	A	F
Glands adrenals	White	Black	G	D
Elements metal wood	White (Co) White (GB)	Red (Lu) Green (Li)	G (Co) G (GB)	C (Lu) A (Li)

Voice loss

Loss of voice.
Ear points: 1, 35, 34, 7.

STEPS	COLORS		SOUNDS	
	V-Out **A-In**	**In** **Out**	**A-Out** **V-In**	**In** **Out**
Area vocal cords	Green	Yellow	A	F
Glands gonads thymus thyroid	White	Black	G	D
Element wood	White (GB)	Green (Li)	G (GB)	A (Li)

The Digestive System

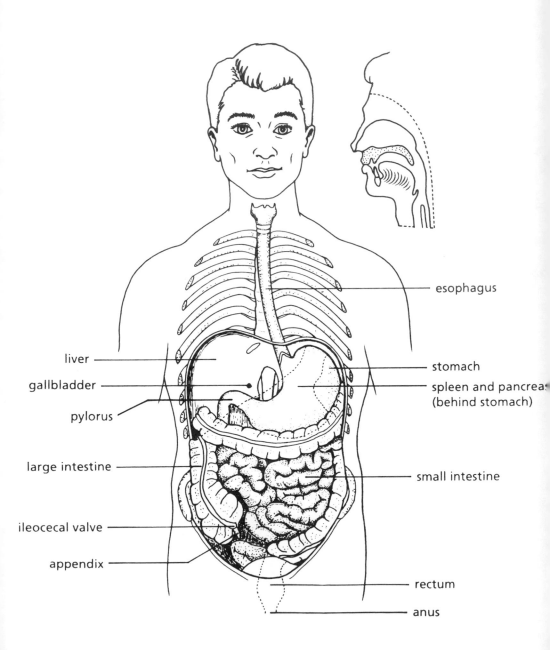

esophagus

liver

gallbladder

pylorus

large intestine

ileocecal valve

appendix

stomach

spleen and pancreas
(behind stomach)

small intestine

rectum

anus

Acid stomach

Excessive amount of hydrochloric acid in the gastric juices, causing heartburn.
Ear points: 35, 6, 21.

STEPS	COLORS		SOUNDS	
	V-Out **A-In**	**In** **Out**	**A-Out** **V-In**	**In** **Out**
Area stomach	Green	Yellow	A	F
Glands pancreas adrenals	White	Black	G	D
Element wood	White (GB)	Green (Li)	G (GB)	A (Li)

Aerophagia, aerocolia, intestinal bloating

Disorders characterized by air trapped in the digestive tract.
Ear points: 26 ext., 6. Add 31 if treating aerocolia.

STEPS	COLORS		SOUNDS	
	V-Out **A-In**	**In** **Out**	**A-Out** **V-In**	**In** **Out**
Area stomach (for aerophagia) colon (for aerocolia) small intestine (for bloating)	Green	Yellow	A	F
Glands pancreas adrenals thyroid	White	Black	G	D
Elements metal fire	White (Co) Blue (SI)	Red (Lu) Red (Ht)	G (Co) D (SI)	C (Lu) C (Ht)

161

Anal fistula

Seek medical attention

Lesion of the anal sphincter, often causing bleeding and itching.
Ear points: 8, 31, 12.

Steps	Colors		Sounds	
	V-Out **A-In**	**In** **Out**	**A-Out** **V-In**	**In** **Out**
Area anus rectum	Green	Yellow	A	F
Glands gonads adrenals thymus	White	Black	G	D
Elements metal wood	White (Co) White (GB)	Red (Lu) Green (Li)	G (Co) G (GB)	C (Lu) A (Li)

Appendicitis

Seek medical attention

Inflammation of the appendix.
Ear points: 35, 6, 31.

Steps	Colors		Sounds	
	V-Out **A-In**	**In** **Out**	**A-Out** **V-In**	**In** **Out**
Area appendix	Green	Yellow	A	F
Glands adrenals thymus	White	Black	G	D
Elements wood metal	White (GB) White (Co)	Green (Li) Red (Lu)	G (GB) G (Co)	A (Li) C (Lu)

Cirrhosis of the liver

Seek medical attention

Liver disease characterized by orange-yellow granules in the liver, hardening of liver tissue, and eventual failure of liver function.
Ear points: 21, 11.

STEPS	COLORS		SOUNDS	
	V-Out **A-In**	**In** **Out**	**A-Out** **V-In**	**In** **Out**
Area liver	Green	Yellow	A	F
Glands entire endo- crine system	White	Black	G	D
Elements wood water	White (GB) Blue (Bl)	Green (Li) Yellow (Ki)	G (GB) D (Bl)	A (Li) F (Ki)

Colic

Strong pain in the abdominal area.
Ear points: 9, 11, 24.

STEPS	COLORS		SOUNDS	
	V-Out **A-In**	**In** **Out**	**A-Out** **V-In**	**In** **Out**
Area abdomen	Green	Yellow	A	F
Glands pancreas adrenals thyroid	White	Black	G	D
Element metal	White (Co)	Red (Lu)	G (Co)	C (Lu)

Colitis

Inflammation of the colon.
Ear points: 35, 21, 31.

STEPS	COLORS		SOUNDS	
	V-Out **A-In**	**In** **Out**	**A-Out** **V-In**	**In** **Out**
Area large intestine	Green	Yellow	A	F
Glands adrenals thymus	White	Black	G	D
Elements				
wood	White (GB)	Green (Li)	G (GB)	A (Li)
metal	White (Co)	Red (Lu)	G (Co)	C (Lu)
water	Blue (Bl)	Yellow (Ki)	D (Bl)	F (Ki)

Constipation

Difficulty with the passage of feces.
Ear points: 21, 11, 31.

STEPS	COLORS		SOUNDS	
	V-Out **A-In**	**In** **Out**	**A-Out** **V-In**	**In** **Out**
Area colon, especially sigmoid flexure	Green	Yellow	A	F
Glands adrenals	White	Black	G	D
Elements				
wood	White (GB)	Green (Li)	G (GB)	A (Li)
metal	White (Co)	Red (Lu)	G (Co)	C (Lu)
water	Blue (Bl)	Yellow (Ki)	D (Bl)	F (Ki)

Diarrhea

Frequent passage of liquid stools.
Ear points: 6, 9, 31, 12.

STEPS	COLORS		SOUNDS	
	V-Out **A-In**	**In** **Out**	**A-Out** **V-In**	**In** **Out**
Area colon, especially ileocecal valve	Green	Yellow	A	F
Glands adrenals	White	Black	G	D
Elements				
wood	White (GB)	Green (Li)	G (GB)	A (Li)
metal	White (Co)	Red (Lu)	G (Co)	C (Lu)

Diverticulitis

Inflammation of a diverticulum (hernia in the wall of the large intestine).
Ear points: 35, 21, 31

STEPS	COLORS		SOUNDS	
	V-Out **A-In**	**In** **Out**	**A-Out** **V-In**	**In** **Out**
Area colon, especially descending colon, sigmoid flexure	Green	Yellow	A	F
Glands adrenals thymus	White	Black	G	D
Elements				
wood	White (GB)	Green (Li)	G (GB)	A (Li)
metal	White (Co)	Red (Lu)	G (Co)	C (Lu)

Flatulence

Accumulation of gas in the intestine, causing abdominal bloating.
Ear points: 26 ext., 6, 31.

STEPS	COLORS		SOUNDS	
	V-Out **A-In**	**In** **Out**	**A-Out** **V-In**	**In** **Out**
Area colon, especially sigmoid flexure	Green	Yellow	A	F
Gland pancreas	White	Black	G	D
Elements				
fire	Blue (SI)	Red (Ht)	D (SI)	C (Ht)
wood	White (GB)	Green (Li)	G (GB)	A (Li)

Gallstones

Seek medical attention

Crystalization of lipid particles, especially cholesterol, in the gallbladder
or biliary passages.
Ear points: 26 ext., 21, 11.

STEPS	COLORS		SOUNDS	
	V-Out **A-In**	**In** **Out**	**A-Out** **V-In**	**In** **Out**
Area gallbladder	Green	Yellow	A	F
Gland thyroid	White	Black	G	D
Element				
wood	White (GB)	Green (Li)	G (GB)	A (Li)

Gastralgia

Sharp stomach pain.
Ear points: 6, 21, 24.

STEPS	COLORS		SOUNDS	
	V-Out **A-In**	**In** **Out**	**A-Out** **V-In**	**In** **Out**
Area stomach	Green	Yellow	A	F
Glands pancreas adrenals	White	Black	G	D
Element wood	White (GB)	Green (Li)	G (GB)	A (Li)

Hemorrhoids

Dilated veins in swollen tissue around the anus or within the rectum.
Ear points: 26 int., 35, 31, 12, 24.

STEPS	COLORS		SOUNDS	
	V-Out **A-In**	**In** **Out**	**A-Out** **V-In**	**In** **Out**
Area rectum	Green	Yellow	A	F
Glands gonads adrenals thymus	White	Black	G	D
Elements metal wood	White (Co) White (GB)	Red (Lu) Green (Li)	G (Co) G (GB)	C (Lu) A (Li)

Hepatitis

Seek medical attention

Inflammation of the liver.
Ear points: 35, 21, 11.

STEPS	COLORS		SOUNDS	
	V-Out **A-In**	**In** **Out**	**A-Out** **V-In**	**In** **Out**
Area liver	Green	Yellow	A	F
Glands adrenals thymus	White	Black	G	D
Elements water metal	Blue (Bl) White (Co)	Yellow (Ki) Red (Lu)	D (Bl) G (Co)	F (Ki) C (Lu)

Hernia

Outpouching of an organ or intrusion of it into another internal space from its normal cavity.
Ear points: Affected area and 9, 11.

STEPS	COLORS		SOUNDS	
	V-Out **A-In**	**In** **Out**	**A-Out** **V-In**	**In** **Out**

Area
groin for
  inguinal hernia
stomach and
  diaphragm for
  hiatus hernia
	Green	Yellow	A	F

Glands adrenals	White	Black	G	D
Element wood	White (GB)	Green (Li)	G (GB)	A (Li)

Indigestion

Temporary abdominal indisposition due to improper or incomplete
digestion.
Ear points: 26 int. and ext., 6, 21, 11.

STEPS	COLORS		SOUNDS	
	V-Out **A-In**	**In** **Out**	**A-Out** **V-In**	**In** **Out**
Area stomach pancreas	Green	Yellow	A	F
Gland pancreas	White	Black	G	D
Elements				
wood	White (GB)	Green (Li)	G (GB)	A (Li)
fire	Blue (SI)	Red (Ht)	D (SI)	C (Ht)
metal	White (Co)	Red (Lu)	G (Co)	C (Lu)

Jaundice

Seek medical attention

Yellowish coloring of the skin and mucous membranes caused by improper processing of bile and the deposition of biliary pigments
in the tissues.
Ear points: 1, 21, 11.

STEPS	COLORS		SOUNDS	
	V-Out **A-In**	**In** **Out**	**A-Out** **V-In**	**In** **Out**
Area hypothalamus	Green	Yellow	A	F
Gland pancreas	White	Black	G	D
Element wood	White (GB)	Green (Li)	G (GB)	A (Li)

Nausea

The urge to vomit.
Ear points: 6, 21, 11; pull the lobe at no. 16.

STEPS	COLORS		SOUNDS	
	V-Out A-In	**In Out**	**A-Out V-In**	**In Out**
Area stomach	Green	Yellow	A	F
Glands pancreas adrenals pituitary	White	Black	G	D
Element wood	White (GB)	Green (Li)	G (GB)	A (Li)

Ulcer

Seek medical attention

Lesion in the mucous membranes of the stomach or duodenum.
Ear points: Affected area and 26 ext., 35, 6, 21.

STEPS	COLORS		SOUNDS	
	V-Out A-In	**In Out**	**A-Out V-In**	**In Out**
Area affected area	Green	Yellow	A	F
Glands adrenals	White	Black	G	D
Elements fire	Blue (SI)	Red (Ht)	D (SI)	C (Ht)
metal	White (Co)	Red (Lu)	G (Co)	C (Lu)

Vomiting

Expulsion of the stomach's contents.
Ear points: 16, 6, 11.

STEPS	COLORS		SOUNDS	
	V-Out **A-In**	**In** **Out**	**A-Out** **V-In**	**In** **Out**
Area stomach	Green	Yellow	Λ	F
Glands pancreas adrenals pituitary	White	Black	G	D
Element wood	White (GB)	Green (Li)	G (GB)	A (Li)

The Urinary System

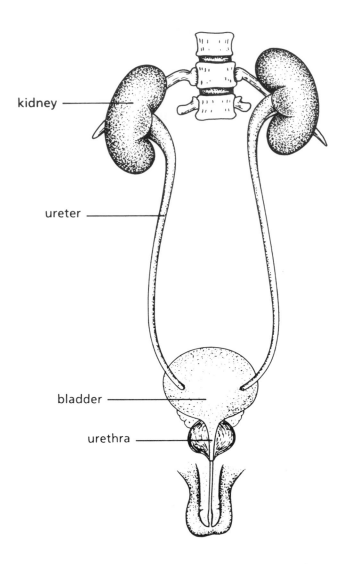

kidney

ureter

bladder

urethra

Cystitis

Inflammation of the bladder.
Ear points: 35, 19 int., 21, 15.

STEPS	COLORS		SOUNDS	
	V-Out **A-In**	**In** **Out**	**A-Out** **V-In**	**In** **Out**
Area bladder	Green	Yellow	A	F
Glands adrenals thymus	White	Black	G	D
Element water	Blue (Bl)	Yellow (Ki)	D (Bl)	F (Ki)

Enuresis, incontinence

Involuntary discharge of urine during sleep or wakefulness.
Ear points: 21, 15, 24.

STEPS	COLORS		SOUNDS	
	V-Out **A-In**	**In** **Out**	**A-Out** **V-In**	**In** **Out**
Area hypothalamus	Green	Yellow	A	F
Glands adrenals pituitary	White	Black	G	D
Element water	Blue (Bl)	Yellow (Ki)	D (Bl)	F (Ki)

Kidney stones

Seek medical attention

Concretion of mineral salts or organic matter in the kidney.
Ear points: 26 int., 35, 21, 15.

STEPS	COLORS		SOUNDS	
	V-Out **A-In**	**In** **Out**	**A-Out** **V-In**	**In** **Out**
Area urinary system	Green	Yellow	A	F
Glands parathyroids pituitary	White	Black	G	D
Element water	Blue (Bl)	Yellow (Ki)	D (Bl)	F (Ki)

Nephritis

Seek medical attention

Inflammation of the kidney.
Ear points: 35, 21, 15.

STEPS	COLORS		SOUNDS	
	V-Out **A-In**	**In** **Out**	**A-Out** **V-In**	**In** **Out**
Area kidney ureter bladder	Green	Yellow	A	F
Glands adrenals thymus	White	Black	G	D
Element wood	White (GB)	Green (Li)	G (GB)	A (Li)

Renal insufficiency

Seek medical attention

Disorder of kidney function.
Ear points: 26 int. and ext., 28, 19 int., 15.

STEPS	COLORS		SOUNDS	
	V-Out **A-In**	**In** **Out**	**A-Out** **V-In**	**In** **Out**
Area hypothalamus	Green	Yellow	A	F
Glands adrenals pituitary	White	Black	G	D
Element water	Blue (Bl)	Yellow (Ki)	D (Bl)	F (Ki)

Uremia

Seek medical attention

Accumulation in the blood of nitrogenous products, generally linked to
serious renal insufficiency.
Ear points: 35, 21, 15.

STEPS	COLORS		SOUNDS	
	V-Out **A-In**	**In** **Out**	**A-Out** **V-In**	**In** **Out**
Area hypothalamus	Green	Yellow	A	F
Glands adrenals pituitary	White	Black	G	`D
Element water	Blue (Bl)	Yellow (Ki)	D (Bl)	F (Ki)

The Sensory Organs

The Mouth and Nose

Cold sore

Viral sore usually located on the lips.
Ear points: Affected area and 26 ext., 11, 24.

STEPS	COLORS		SOUNDS	
	V-Out **A-In**	**In** **Out**	**A-Out** **V-In**	**In** **Out**
Area affected area	Green	Yellow	A	F
Glands adrenals thymus	White	Black	G	D
Element wood	White (GB)	Green (Li)	G (GB)	A (Li)

Halitosis

Strong bad breath.
Ear points: 6, 9, 11, 31.

STEPS	COLORS		SOUNDS	
	V-Out **A-In**	**In** **Out**	**A-Out** **V-In**	**In** **Out**
Area mouth	Green	Yellow	A	F
Glands pancreas thyroid	White	Black	G	D
Elements wood	White (GB)	Green (Li)	G (GB)	A (Li)
fire	Blue (SI)	Red (Ht)	D (SI)	C(Ht)
metal	White (Co)	Red (Lu)	G (Co)	C (Lu)

Loss of taste and smell

Inability to properly distinguish flavors and odors.
Ear points: 1, 2, 5, 7.

STEPS	COLORS		SOUNDS	
	V-Out **A-In**	**In** **Out**	**A-Out** **V-In**	**In** **Out**
Area nasal mucous membrane tongue	Green	Yellow	A	F
Glands gonads pancreas	White	Black	G	D
Element metal	White (Co)	Red (Lu)	G (Co)	C (Lu)

Mumps

Contagious disease characterized by an inflammation of the parotid
gland.
Ear points: 1, 35, 5 .

STEPS	COLORS		SOUNDS	
	V-Out **A-In**	**In** **Out**	**A-Out** **V-In**	**In** **Out**
Area affected area	Green	Yellow	A	F
Glands adrenals thymus thyroid	White	Black	G	D
Elements fire wood	Blue (SI) White(GB)	Red (Ht) Green (Li)	D (SI) G (GB)	C (Ht) A (Li)

Nosebleed

Abnormal flow of blood from the nasal walls.
Ear points: 2, 9, 11. It also helps to place a cold facecloth on the back of
 the neck.

Steps	Colors		Sounds	
	V-Out A-In	**In Out**	**A-Out V-In**	**In Out**
Area nose	Green	Yellow	A	F
Glands adrenals gonads pancreas	White	Black	G	D
Element water	Blue (Bl)	Yellow (Ki)	D (Bl)	F (Ki)

Nose polyp

Growth, generally benign, of the nasal mucous membrane.
Ear points: 1, 2, 11.

Steps	Colors		Sounds	
	V-Out A-In	**In Out**	**A-Out V-In**	**In Out**
Area nose	Green	Yellow	A	F
Glands adrenals thymus pituitary	White	Black	G	D
Element metal	White (Co)	Red (Lu)	G (Co)	C (Lu)

Pyorrhea

Purulent inflammation of tooth sockets, causing teeth to loosen.
Ear points: 1, 3, 6, 21.

STEPS	COLORS		SOUNDS	
	V-Out **A-In**	**In** **Out**	**A-Out** **V-In**	**In** **Out**
Area gums	Green	Yellow	A	F
Glands adrenals thymus pituitary	White	Black	G	D
Element wood	White (GB)	Green(Li)	G (GB)	A (Li)

Stomatitis

Inflammation of the mucous membrane of the mouth.
Ear points: 1,17, 35, 3, 11.

STEPS	COLORS		SOUNDS	
	V-Out **A-In**	**In** **Out**	**A-Out** **V-In**	**In** **Out**
Area mouth	Green	Yellow	A	F
Glands adrenals thymus	White	Black	G	D
Element fire wood	Blue (SI) White (GB)	Red (Ht) Green (Li)	D (SI) G (GB)	C (Ht) A (Li)

179

Toothache

Pain in the teeth and gums.
Ear points: 1, 3, 17, 11, 26 int. and ext.

STEPS	COLORS		SOUNDS	
	V-Out **A-In**	**In** **Out**	**A-Out** **V-In**	**In** **Out**
Area affected area	Green	Yellow	A	F
Glands thymus pituitary	White	Black	G	D
Elements water metal	Blue (Bl) White (Co)	Yellow (Ki) Red (Lu)	D (Bl) G (Co)	F (Ki) C (Lu)

The Eyes

Atrophy of the optic nerve

Seek medical attention

Degeneration of the fibers of the optic nerve, accompanied by impaired
  vision.
Ear points: 16, 1, 21, 9, 11.

STEPS	COLORS		SOUNDS	
	V-Out **A-In**	**In** **Out**	**A-Out** **V-In**	**In** **Out**
Area optic nerve	Green	Yellow	A	F
Glands adrenals pituitary	White	Black	G	D
Element wood	White (GB)	Green (Li)	G (GB)	A (Li)

Cataract

Seek medical attention

Clouding of the eye's crystalline lens.
Ear points: 1, 35, 15.

STEPS	COLORS		SOUNDS	
	V-Out **A-In**	**In** **Out**	**A-Out** **V-In**	**In** **Out**
Area lens of the eye	Green	Yellow	A	F
Glands adrenals thymus pituitary	White	Black	G	D
Element water	Blue (Bl)	Yellow (Ki)	D (Bl)	F (Ki)

Chalazion

Circumscribed swelling in the lid caused by the chronic inflammation
and obstruction of a lid gland.
Ear points: 1, 35, 33, 11.

STEPS	COLORS		SOUNDS	
	V-Out **A-In**	**In** **Out**	**A-Out** **V-In**	**In** **Out**
Area eyelid	Green	Yellow	A	F
Glands adrenals pituitary	White	Black	G	D
Element water wood	Blue (Bl) White (GB)	Yellow (Ki) Green (Li)	D (Bl) G (GB)	F (Ki) A (Li)

Conjunctivitis

Inflammation of the membranes lining the eyes and lids.
Ear points: 1, 35, 11, 24.

Steps	Colors		Sounds	
	V-Out A-In	In Out	A-Out V-In	In Out
Area inside of the eye and lids	Green	Yellow	A	F
Glands adrenals thymus	White	Black	G	D
Element water wood	Blue (Bl) White (GB)	Yellow (Ki) Green (Li)	D (Bl) G (GB)	F (Ki) A (Li)

Detached retina

Seek medical attention

Partial or complete separation of the retina from the choroid layer.
Ear points: 1, 35, 11.

Steps	Colors		Sounds	
	V-Out A-In	In Out	A-Out V-In	In Out
Area retina choroid	Green	Yellow	A	F
Glands adrenals thyroid pituitary	White	Black	G	D
Element wood	White (GB)	Green (Li)	G (GB)	A (Li)

Eye fatigue

Smarting or burning sensation in the eyes.
Ear points: 1, 21, 24.

STEPS	COLORS		SOUNDS	
	V-Out A-In	**In Out**	**A-Out V-In**	**In Out**
Area eyes	Green	Yellow	A	F
Glands adrenals thymus thyroid	White	Black	G	D
Element wood	White (GB)	Green (Li)	G (GB)	A (Li)

Glaucoma

Seek medical attention

Build up of excessive pressure in the liquid inside the eyeball.
Ear points: 1, 35, 15.

STEPS	COLORS		SOUNDS	
	V-Out A-In	**In Out**	**A-Out V-In**	**In Out**
Area eyeball	Green	Yellow	A	F
Glands adrenals pituitary	White	Black	G	D
Element water	Blue (Bl)	Yellow (Ki)	D (Bl)	F (Ki)

Iritis

Seek medical attention

Inflammation of the iris.
Ear points: 1, 35, 11, 24.

STEPS	COLORS		SOUNDS	
	V-Out **A-In**	**In** **Out**	**A-Out** **V-In**	**In** **Out**
Area iris	Green	Yellow	A	F
Glands adrenals thymus	White	Black	G	D
Element wood	White (GB)	Green (Li)	G (GB)	A (Li)

Ophthalmic shingles

Seek medical attention

Viral infection in the eye, causing sharp pain.
Ear points: 16, 1, 21.

STEPS	COLORS		SOUNDS	
	V-Out **A-In**	**In** **Out**	**A-Out** **V-In**	**In** **Out**
Area eye	Green	Yellow	A	F
Glands adrenals thymus	White	Black	G	D
Element wood	White (GB)	Green (Li)	G (GB)	A (Li)

Sty

Small purulent localized infection along the edge of the eyelid.
Ear points: 1, 35, 11, 24.

STEPS	COLORS		SOUNDS	
	V-Out **A-In**	**In** **Out**	**A-Out** **V-In**	**In** **Out**
Area eyelid	Green	Yellow	A	F
Glands adrenals thymus	White	Black	G	D
Element wood	White (GB)	Green (Li)	G (GB)	A (Li)

The Ears

Buzzing in the ears

Ringing, whistling, or other unusual sounds inside the ear, caused by
  physiological problems (accumulated wax, wisdom teeth in poor
  condition, blocked Eustachian tubes, etc.).
Ear points: Massage along the entire distance separating points 28 and
  29, 5, 11, 15.

STEPS	COLORS		SOUNDS	
	V-Out **A-In**	**In** **Out**	**A-Out** **V-In**	**In** **Out**
Area ears	Green	Yellow	A	F
Glands adrenals thymus pineal	White	Black	G	D
Element fire	Blue (SI)	Red (Ht)	D (SI)	C (Ht)
water	Blue (Bl)	Yellow (Ki)	D (Bl)	F (Ki)
wood	White (GB)	Green (Li)	G (GB)	A (Li)

Deafness

Seek medical attention

Partial or complete loss of hearing.

Ear points: 1, 19 ext. and areas behind the ears.

STEPS	COLORS		SOUNDS	
	V-Out A-In	In Out	A-Out V-In	In Out
Area ears	Green	Yellow	A	F
Glands pancreas thyroid	White	Black	G	D
Element water	Blue (Bl)	Yellow (Ki)	D (Bl)	F (Ki)

Motion sickness

Nausea, vomiting, or dizziness caused by the movement of a vehicle.

Ear points: Massage along the entire distance separating points 28 and 29, 21.

STEPS	COLORS		SOUNDS	
	V-Out A-In	In Out	A-Out V-In	In Out
Area middle and inner ear	Green	Yellow	A	F
Glands pancreas adrenals pineal	White	Black	G	D
Elements water wood	Blue (Bl) White (GB)	Yellow (Ki) Green (Li)	D (Bl) G (GB)	F (Ki) A (Li)

Otalgia

Seek medical attention

Earache from any of several causes. Check for dental cavities, tongue
injury or sore, throat ailment.

Ear points: 1, 5, 20, 24.

STEPS	COLORS		SOUNDS	
	V-Out **A-In**	**In** **Out**	**A-Out** **V-In**	**In** **Out**
Area ears	Green	Yellow	A	F
Glands adrenals thymus pituitary	White	Black	G	D
Element water	Blue (Bl)	Yellow (Ki)	D (Bl)	F (Ki)

Otitis

Seek medical attention

Acute or chronic inflammation of the ear.

Ear points: 1, 5, 20, 24.

STEPS	COLORS		SOUNDS	
	V-Out **A-In**	**In** **Out**	**A-Out** **V-In**	**In** **Out**
Area ears	Green	Yellow	A	F
Glands adrenals thymus pituitary	White	Black	G	D
Elements water wood	Blue (Bl) White (GB)	Yellow (Ki) Green (Li)	D (Bl) G (GB)	F (Ki) A (Li)

187

The Skin

Acne

Skin eruption caused by inflammation of the skin glands and hair follicles.

Ear points: 16, 19 int., 21, 11, 24.

STEPS	COLORS		SOUNDS	
	V-Out **A-In**	**In** **Out**	**A-Out** **V-In**	**In** **Out**
Area affected area	Green	Yellow	A	F
Glands gonads adrenals thyroid	White	Black	G	D
Elements metal	White (Co)	Red (Lu)	G (Co)	C (Lu)
water	Blue (Bl)	Yellow (Ki)	D (Bl)	F (Ki)
wood	White (GB)	Green (Li)	G (GB)	A (Li)

Burns, sunburns, cuts, stings

Skin injury caused by excessive sun or heat, sharp edges, or insects.

Ear points: 1, 19 int., 35.

STEPS	COLORS		SOUNDS	
	V-Out **A-In**	**In** **Out**	**A-Out** **V-In**	**In** **Out**
Area affected area	Green	Yellow	A	F
Glands adrenals thymus pituitary	White	Black	G	D
Element metal	White (Co)	Red (Lu)	G (Co)	C (Lu)

188

Dry skin

Persistence of a layer of dry, dead cells on the skin as a result of a
slowing of cellular regeneration.
Ear points: 26 ext., 19 int., 15, 24.

STEPS	COLORS		SOUNDS	
	V-Out **A-In**	**In** **Out**	**A-Out** **V-In**	**In** **Out**
Area affected area	Green	Yellow	A	F
Glands gonads adrenals thyroid	White	Black	G	D
Elements metal wood	White (Co) White (GB)	Red (Lu) Green (Li)	G (Co) G (GB)	C (Lu) A (Li)

Eczema

Skin condition characterized by redness and oozing vesicular lesions.
Ear points: 26 int., 19 int., 15, 24.

STEPS	COLORS		SOUNDS	
	V-Out **A-In**	**In** **Out**	**A-Out** **V-In**	**In** **Out**
Area affected area	Green	Yellow	A	F
Glands adrenals thymus thyroid	White	Black	G	D
Elements metal wood	White (Co) White (GB)	Red (Lu) Green (Li)	G (Co) G (GB)	C (Lu) A (Li)

Excessive perspiration

Overly abundant perspiration.
Ear points: 26 ext., 21, 15.

Steps	Colors		Sounds	
	V-Out **A-In**	**In** **Out**	**A-Out** **V-In**	**In** **Out**
Area affected area	Green	Yellow	A	F
Glands adrenals thyroid	White	Black	G	D
Element water	Blue (Bl)	Yellow (Ki)	D (Bl)	F (Ki)

Hives (urticaria)

Raised edematous patches of skin or mucous membrane, usually caused
by an allergy.
Ear points: 26 ext., 19 int., 11, 24.

Steps	Colors		Sounds	
	V-Out **A-In**	**In** **Out**	**A-Out** **V-In**	**In** **Out**
Area affected area	Green	Yellow	A	F
Glands adrenals	White	Black	G	D
Element metal	White (Co)	Red (Lu)	G (Co)	C (Lu)

190

Psoriasis

Skin disease characterized by red patches covered with an abundance of white scales, especially on the elbows, knees, and scalp.

Ear points: 26 int., 19 int., 11, 21.

STEPS	COLORS		SOUNDS	
	V-Out **A-In**	**In** **Out**	**A-Out** **V-In**	**In** **Out**
Area affected area	Green	Yellow	A	F
Glands gonads adrenals thyroid	White	Black	G	D
Elements				
wood	White (GB)	Green (Li)	G (GB)	A (Li)
metal	White (Co)	Red (Lu)	G (Co)	C (Lu)
water	Blue (Bl)	Yellow (Ki)	D (Bl)	F (Ki)

Shingles

Seek medical attention

Illness of viral origin characterized by vesicular eruption and pain along the track of specific sensory nerves.

Ear points: Affected area and 21.

STEPS:	COLORS		SOUNDS	
	V-Out **A-In**	**In** **Out**	**A-Out** **V-In**	**In** **Out**
Area affected area	Green	Yellow	A	F
Glands adrenals thymus pituitary	White	Black	G	D
Element wood	White (GB)	Green (Li)	G (GB)	A (Li)

Ulcer

Seek medical attention

Lesion of the skin or mucous membrane that does not heal normally.
Ear points: Affected area and 1, 21.

STEPS	COLORS		SOUNDS	
	V-Out **A-In**	**In** **Out**	**A-Out** **V-In**	**In** **Out**
Area affected area	Green	Yellow	A	F
Glands adrenals pituitary	White	Black	G	D
Element metal	White (Co)	Red (Lu)	G (Co)	C (Lu)

Vitiligo

Altered pigmentation characterized by smooth white patches on different areas of the body.
Ear points: 26 ext., 19 int., 21, 11.

STEPS	COLORS		SOUNDS	
	V-Out **A-In**	**In** **Out**	**A-Out** **V-In**	**In** **Out**
Area affected area	Green	Yellow	A	F
Glands adrenals pineal	White	Black	G.	D
Element wood	White (GB)	Green (Li)	G (GB)	A (Li)

Warts, cysts, tumors

Seek medical attention

Growths caused by abnormal proliferation of cells.
Ear points: 1, 8, 11, 15.

STEPS	COLORS		SOUNDS	
	V-Out **A-In**	**In** **Out**	**A-Out** **V-In**	**In** **Out**
Area affected area	Green	Yellow	A	F
Glands gonads pituitary	White	Black	G	D
Element wood	White (GB)	Green (Li)	G (GB)	A (Li)

The Reproductive System

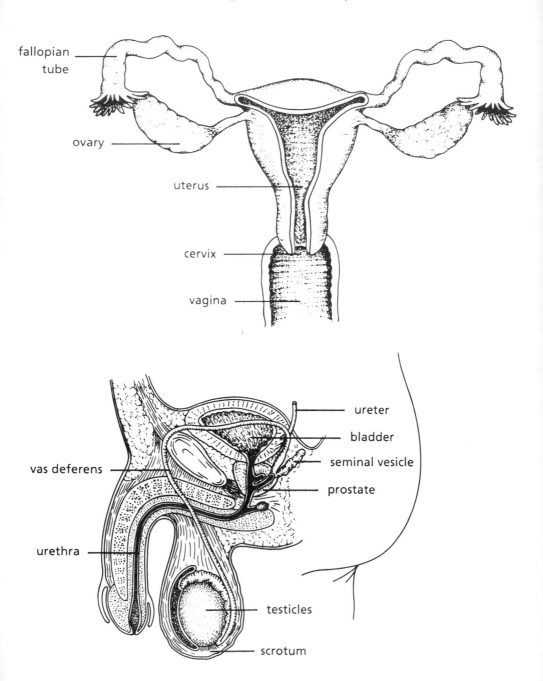

Amenorrhea

Absence of menstral flow in a woman of menstruating age.
Ear points: 17, 26 int., 29, 8.

STEPS	COLORS		SOUNDS	
	V-Out **A-In**	**In** **Out**	**A-Out** **V-In**	**In** **Out**
Area hypothalamus	Green	Yellow	A	F
Glands gonads adrenals pituitary	White	Black	G	D
Elements fire wood	Blue (SI) White (GB)	Red (Ht) Green (Li)	D (SI) G (GB)	C (Ht) A (Li)

Childbirth

Passage of an infant from the mother's uterus into the outer world.
Ear points: 17, 8, 12.

STEPS	COLORS		SOUNDS	
	V-Out **A-In**	**In** **Out**	**A-Out** **V-In**	**In** **Out**
Area uterus	Green	Yellow	A	F
Glands ovaries adrenals pituitary	White	Black	G	D
Elements fire wood	Blue (SI) White (GB)	Red (Ht) Green (Li)	D (SI) G (GB)	C (Ht) A (Li)

Congested breasts

Swelling of the lymph glands in the breasts.
Ear points: 19 int., 21, 8.

STEPS	COLORS		SOUNDS	
	V-Out **A-In**	**In** **Out**	**A-Out** **V-In**	**In** **Out**
Area breasts	Green	Yellow	A	F
Glands ovaries adrenals pituitary	White	Black	G	D
Elements fire	Blue (SI)	Red (Ht)	D (SI)	C (Ht)
wood	White (GB)	Green (Li)	G (GB)	A (Li)

Cysts on the ovaries or breasts

Seek medical attention

Pathological growths on the ovaries or in the breasts.
Ear points: 3, 29, 8, 15.

STEPS	COLORS		SOUNDS	
	V-Out **A-In**	**In** **Out**	**A-Out** **V-In**	**In** **Out**
Area ovaries or breasts	Green	Yellow	A	F
Glands thymus pituitary	White	Black	G	D
Element wood	White (GB)	Green (Li)	G (GB)	A (Li)

Dysmenorrhea

Painful menstrual periods.
Ear points: 17, 26 int., 29, 8.

STEPS	COLORS		SOUNDS	
	V-Out **A-In**	**In** **Out**	**A-Out** **V-In**	**In** **Out**
Area painful area	Green	Yellow	A	F
Glands ovaries parathyroids pituitary	White	Black	G	D
Elements				
fire	Blue (SI)	Red (Ht)	D (SI)	C (Ht)
water	Blue (Bl)	Yellow (Ki)	D (Bl)	F (Ki)
wood	White (GB)	Green (Li)	G (GB)	A (Li)

Fibroma

Seek medical attention

Tumor of the uterus formed by fibrous tissue.
Ear points: 17, 26 int., 29, 8.

STEPS	COLORS		SOUNDS	
	V-Out **A-In**	**In** **Out**	**A-Out** **V-In**	**In** **Out**
Area uterus	Green	Yellow	A	F
Glands ovaries pancreas pituitary	White	Black	G	D
Elements				
fire	Blue (SI)	Red (Ht)	D (SI)	C (Ht)
wood	White (GB)	Green (Li)	G (GB)	A (Li)

Hot flashes

Transitory sensations of heat, a normal symptom in women reaching
menopause.
Ear points: 17, 26 int., 29, 8.

STEPS	COLORS		SOUNDS	
	V-Out **A-In**	**In** **Out**	**A-Out** **V-In**	**In** **Out**
Area hypothalamus	Green	Yellow	A	F
Glands ovaries adrenals pituitary	White	Black	G	D
Elements fire	Blue (SI)	Red (Ht)	D (SI)	C (Ht)
wood	White (GB)	Green (Li)	G (GB)	A (Li)

Hysterectomy

Removal of the uterus, sometimes including the ovaries and fallopian
tubes.
Ear points: 29, 35, 21.

STEPS	COLORS		SOUNDS	
	V-Out **A-In**	**In** **Out**	**A-Out** **V-In**	**In** **Out**
Area uterus ovaries fallopian tubes	Green	Yellow	A	F
Glands adrenals thyroid pituitary	White	Black	G	D
Elements fire	Blue (SI)	Red (Ht)	D (SI)	C (Ht)
water	Blue (Bl)	Yellow (Ki)	D (Bl)	F (Ki)
wood	White (GB)	Green (Li)	G (GB)	A (Li)

Impotence

Physical inability of a man to copulate.
Ear points: 29, 21, 8.

STEPS	COLORS		SOUNDS	
	V-Out A-In	**In Out**	**A-Out V-In**	**In Out**
Area hypothalamus	Green	Yellow	A	F
Glands testicles adrenals pituitary	White	Black	G	D
Elements fire	Blue (SI)	Red (Ht)	D (SI)	C (Ht)
water	Blue (Bl)	Yellow (Ki)	D (Bl)	F (Ki)

Infertility

Dysfunction of the reproductive organs from any of several causes, such as blocked fallopian tubes, irregular ovulation, suppressed libido, or low sperm count.
Ear points: 21, 17, 26 int., 29, 8.

STEPS	COLORS		SOUNDS	
	V-Out A-In	**In Out**	**A-Out V-In**	**In Out**
Area in women, ovaries, fallopian tubes, uterus in men, testicles, vas deferens, prostate	Green	Yellow	A	F
Glands gonads adrenals pituitary	White	Black	G	D
Elements fire	Blue (SI)	Red (Ht)	D (SI)	C (Ht)
wood	White (GB)	Green (Li)	G (GB)	A (Li)

Leukorrhea

Whitish, occasionally purulent vaginal discharge.
Ear points: 27, 24, 8.

STEPS	COLORS		SOUNDS	
	V-Out **A-In**	**In** **Out**	**A-Out** **V-In**	**In** **Out**
Area vagina vulva	Green	Yellow	A	F
Glands ovaries thyroid pituitary	White	Black	G	D
Elements fire	Blue (SI)	Red (Ht)	D (SI)	C (Ht)
water	Blue (Bl)	Yellow (Ki)	D (Bl)	F (Ki)

Mastitis

Inflammation of the mammary glands.
Ear points: 29, 35, 21.

STEPS	COLORS		SOUNDS	
	V-Out **A-In**	**In** **Out**	**A-Out** **V-In**	**In** **Out**
Area breasts	Green	Yellow	A	F
Glands adrenals thymus pituitary	White	Black	G	D
Element wood	White (GB)	Green (Li)	G (GB)	A (Li)

Menopause

The cessation of ovulation and menstruation.
Ear points: 29, 21, 8.

STEPS	COLORS		SOUNDS	
	V-Out **A-In**	**In** **Out**	**A-Out** **V-In**	**In** **Out**
Area hypothalamus	Green	Yellow	A	F
Glands entire endo-crine system	White	Black	G	D
Elements				
water	Blue (Bl)	Yellow (Ki)	D (Bl)	F (Ki)
wood	White (GB)	Green (Li)	G (GB)	A (Li)

Menstrual cramps

Abdominal cramps associated with the menstrual period.
Ear points: 28, 19 int., 22. It also helps to squeeze the tongue between
the lips.

STEPS	COLORS		SOUNDS	
	V-Out **A-In**	**In** **Out**	**A-Out** **V-In**	**In** **Out**
Area painful area	Green	Yellow	A	F
Glands ovaries parathyroids pituitary	White	Black	G	D
Elements				
fire	Blue (SI)	Red (Ht)	D (SI)	C (Ht)
water	Blue (Bl)	Yellow (Ki)	D (Bl)	F (Ki)
wood	White (GB)	Green (Li)	G (GB)	A (Li)

Nursing

Feeding of breast milk to an infant.
Ear points: 27, 21, 8.

STEPS	COLORS		SOUNDS	
	V-Out **A-In**	**In** **Out**	**A-Out** **V-In**	**In** **Out**
Area hypothalamus	Green	Yellow	A	F
Glands ovaries pituitary	White	Black	G	D
Element fire	Blue (SI)	Red (Ht)	D (SI)	C (Ht)

Pregnancy-related problems

Generally, nausea and edema.
Ear points: 1, 17, 20, 21, 11, 25, 24. **Do not engage point 27.**

STEPS	COLORS		SOUNDS	
	V-Out **A-In**	**In** **Out**	**A-Out** **V-In**	**In** **Out**
Area painful area	Green	Yellow	A	F
Glands ovaries pancreas pituitary	White	Black	G	D
Elements water	Blue (Bl)	Yellow (Ki)	D (Bl)	F (Ki)
wood	White (GB)	Green (Li)	G (GB)	A (Li)

Prostate problems

Seek medical attention

Generally, inflammation and enlargement of the prostate, resulting in frequent and/or painful urination.
Ear points: 26 int, 35, 8.

STEPS	COLORS		SOUNDS	
	V-Out **A-In**	**In** **Out**	**A-Out** **V-In**	**In** **Out**
Area prostate	Green	Yellow	A	F
Glands testicles adrenals pituitary	White	Black	G	D
Elements water wood	Blue (Bl) White (GB)	Yellow (Ki) Green (Li)	D (Bl) G (GB)	F (Ki) A (Li)

Sexual problems in men

Reduced sex drive or premature ejaculation, often due to physical or mental fatigue.
Ear points: 35, 34, 7.

STEPS	COLORS		SOUNDS	
	V-Out **A-In**	**In** **Out**	**A-Out** **V-In**	**In** **Out**
Area hypothalamus	Green	Yellow	A	F
Glands testicles adrenals pituitary	White	Black	G	D
Elements fire water	Blue (SI) Blue (Bl)	Red (Ht) Yellow (Ki)	D (SI) D (Bl)	C (Ht) F (Ki)

Sexual problems in women

Difficulty in reaching orgasm; vaginismus (painful spasmodic contraction of the vaginal muscles).
Ear points: 29, 3, 7, 8, 12.

STEPS	COLORS		SOUNDS	
	V-Out **A-In**	**In** **Out**	**A-Out** **V-In**	**In** **Out**
Area clitoris vagina	Green	Yellow	A	F
Glands gonads adrenals pituitary	White	Black	G	D
Elements fire wood	Blue (SI) White (GB)	Red (Ht) Green (Li)	D (SI) G (GB)	C (Ht) A (Li)

Tubal ligation–related problems

Hormonal imbalance causing nausea or headaches.
Ear points: 29, 33, 27, 28, 8, 12.

STEPS	COLORS		SOUNDS	
	V-Out **A-In**	**In** **Out**	**A-Out** **V-In**	**In** **Out**
Area fallopian tubes	Green	Yellow	A	F
Glands ovaries pituitary	White	Black	G	D
Elements fire wood	Blue (SI) White (GB)	Red (Ht) Green (Li)	D (SI) G (GB)	C (Ht) A (Li)

8

Harmonizing
the Meridians

All of the body's meridians can be affected by our emotional reactions, but the stomach meridian is the one that absorbs most of the aftershocks, since it must "digest" the events we experience. Disruption of this meridian can lead to phobic states—persistent and excessive fear of particular objects, actions, situations, ideas, animals, or people. According to California psychologist Roger J. Calahan, 95 percent of phobias affect the stomach meridian and the remaining 5 percent affect the liver meridian. He also states that about 20 percent of all people suffer from a variety of phobias: some fear heights, crowds, dentists, doctors, insects, or mice; others are afraid of driving, public speaking, tests, and other activities.[14]

Fear in itself is not bad: we should be prudent when crossing the street; we should live with considerable respect for fire and water; we should prepare properly for interviews. Fear becomes a phobia only when it paralyzes us, preventing us from acting constructively and causing us to retreat within ourselves. The more intense our fear and the more it inhibits action, the more serious is our condition. Phobias mani-

---

14. See Roger J. Calahan, *The Five-Minute Phobia Cure* (Wilmington, Del.: Enterprise Publishing Inc., 1980, 1985) 32, 36, 69, 76.

fest themselves in the meridian network, specifically in the stomach meridian, as a problem of energy distribution.

Correcting Phobias

Since so many people suffer to some extent from phobias, I felt it important to outline a method for correcting this condition. It is a simple, natural, and pain-free technique that applies foot reflexology to a pressure point corresponding to the stomach meridian, often yielding immediate and lasting results. You can practice this technique on yourself or with someone else. (Be sure to trim your nails before working with these pressure points.) Even if you don't have a phobia, try it anyway—it will make you feel bright-eyed and relaxed.

Before you begin, ask yourself or the person you are dealing with to rate the phobia on a scale of one to ten, with ten being the most severe (see the rating scale below). Remember this number, as it will allow you to assess the degree of improvement following the treatments.

When confronted with my fear,

10. I panic. I feel as awful as anyone possibly can.
9. The discomfort is almost unbearable.
8. My fear is very great.
7. My fear is considerable.
6. My fear is a major inconvenience.
5. My fear is an inconvenience, but it's manageable.
4. My fear is annoying, but it's manageable.
3. I'm a bit frightened, but I have the situation under control.
2. I am relatively calm and relaxed, and I have no fear.
1. I am perfectly calm and perfectly relaxed.

Like all other meridians, the meridian of the stomach is bilateral, and it responds differently in the visual and the auditory. The right stomach meridian tends to be overcharged in the visual and undercharged in the auditory. Conversely, the left meridian is likely to be overcharged in the auditory and undercharged in the visual. For a visual, work on the right foot first and finish with the left. When treating an auditory person, begin with the left foot and end with the right.

Right Foot

Inhale deeply. While exhaling, press with the thumb on the outer bottom edge of the nail of the second toe (see figure 18). Repeat three times. Next, ask the person to count for the duration of your exhale (aloud for a visual, silently for an auditory) while you again press the second toe. Repeat this action one more time, asking the person to look down and to the right as you press the toe.

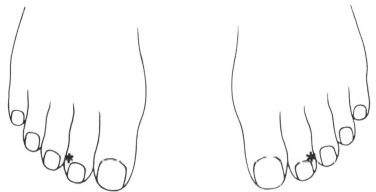

FIGURE 18: Tip of the Stomach Meridian

Left Foot

Inhale deeply. While exhaling, tap on the outer bottom edge of the nail of the second toe with your index and middle fingers. Repeat three times. Next, ask the person to hum (aloud for an auditory, to himself for a visual) as you tap the toe. Finally, ask the person to look down and to the left as you tap the toe.

To obtain the intended results with this technique, it is essential to breathe properly. Remember that inhalation is a time of rest and exhalation is a time of action. Massage, tap, hum, and count only during exhalation.

It is a good idea to inquire between steps as to how the person rates his phobia. He can gauge this instinctively, as the fear exists even in the absence of the phobic trigger. After the third step, he should be able to rate the phobia between levels 3 and 1. At that point, the technique has achieved its desired effect. To confirm this, the person should face his phobic trigger as soon as possible. This can be easy to arrange in some cases, such as a fear of water. In others—the fear of flying, for instance—it may be more difficult. If the person encounters his phobic trigger and is not in a position to confront his fear immediately with this technique, I advise the visual to place his left hand (soothing hand) on his stomach and the auditory to place his right hand (stimulating hand) on his stomach. This will reinforce the corrective action to the stomach meridian, if needed. (I refer specifically to the stomach here, not the belly. If you are uncertain as to the location of the stomach, refer to the figure on page 160.)

If at first this technique seems not to succeed, check to be sure you are breathing fully. Shallow breathing is the main cause of failure. In my experience, this procedure frees 85 percent of all recipients of their phobias. The remaining 15 percent may be victims of a psychological inversion characterized by a negative attitude toward life in general. This inversion can be more or less severe and may be caused by an unconscious self-destructive impulse likely to sabotage any attempt at improving health. It can also be caused by medications such as sedatives, tranquilizers, stimulants, and birth control pills, all of which affect the nervous system.

There is a simple way to stop this inversion long enough to give you time to correct the phobia. If you are a visual, on an exhalation, tap vigorously three times on the little-finger side of the right hand, then three times on the little-finger side of the left hand. This massages the meridian of the small intestine—the body's center of gravity—restoring its energy balance. If you are an auditory, begin by tapping the left hand, then tap three times on the right hand. Follow immediately with the phobia correction technique described above.

This technique can also be used on other meridians to help us face a great many painful situations (figure 19). To help deal with grief and mourning, you must restore the balance of the kidney meridian. The massage point suggested in this instance is on the inside of the small toe. (Although the traditional end point of the kidney meridian is on the sole of the foot, the toe point is more appropriate for this technique.) In dealing with material loss, the large intestine is often involved. The point to massage in this instance is on the inside of the index finger. In the aftermath of a broken heart, an abortion, or rape, the master of the heart meridian is often the one affected. Its point is on the inside of the middle finger.

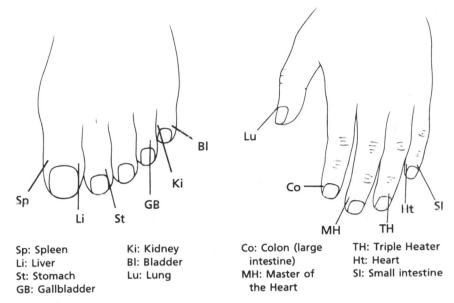

Sp: Spleen   Ki: Kidney   Co: Colon (large   TH: Triple Heater
Li: Liver   Bl: Bladder   intestine)   Ht: Heart
St: Stomach   Lu: Lung   MH: Master of   SI: Small intestine
GB: Gallbladder   the Heart

FIGURE 19: Correspondences Between Meridians and Extremities

Generally, when you experience a strong emotion and you are not certain which meridian is involved, find the finger or toe that is most painful when massaged and apply the steps for phobia correction to that particular finger or toe. Follow with treatment of the same finger or toe on the other hand or foot. You will most likely find this procedure beneficial.

These are the elemental correspondences and attributes for each of the major meridians in the body:

• The **colon** and **lung** meridians, associated with metal, relate to order, caution, and saving. These meridians are helpful in dealing with sadness, depression, and financial loss.

• The **kidney** and **bladder** meridians, associated with water, relate to courage and willpower. These meridians help in times of fear, mourning, or sentimental loss.

• The **liver** and **gallbladder** meridians, associated with wood, relate to imagination and dynamism. These meridians help dissipate anger and bitterness.

• The **small intestine** and **heart** meridians, as well as the **triple warmer** and the **master of the heart**, are associated with fire and relate to wisdom and joy. These meridians are helpful in treating anxiety, overexcitement, and sexual trauma.

• The **stomach** and **spleen** meridians, associated with earth, relate to reflection, memory, and concentration. These meridians are good for dealing with fixed ideas, loss of memory, and anguish.

Obviously, no one's life unfolds without trials or setbacks. Reacting constructively to surprising or painful events can change our life and serve as the springboard to further self-development. Yet we often don't know how to change our habitual reactions or to respond to traumas in a truly life-enriching way.

Harmonizing the meridians restores inner balance, minimizing the effects of distressing events and helping us to be at peace with ourselves and to regain physical and mental health. If you receive a physical or emotional shock, you should immediately employ the preceding techniques to lessen or eliminate the harmful consequences.

Conclusion

While the scope of this book is far-reaching, I don't, by any stretch of the imagination, pretend that the methods presented here can solve all problems. All of us are called to experience situations over which we have little control (mourning, separation, illness, etc.). However, we can face these experiences with greater serenity by using some of the techniques described in this book. These are designed to help us rid ourselves of psychological "knots" by fostering the free flow of energy throughout our entire being.

I find it fascinating to explore the division of humanity into two groups: visuals and auditories. Yet, it seems obvious and incontestible that the two, far from being opposed to each other, are actually complementary—they communicate to each other their approach to the universe and help each other understand life, making it richer, fuller, and more harmonious.

Index

Page numbers for *specific health conditions* are in italics